HOW TO GET STARTED WITH THE VITILIGO DIET

A Beginner's Quick Start Guide to Support Skin Health, Maintain Pigmentation, and Promote Melanin Synthesis

Chris Preston, RDN

ACKNOWLEDGEMENTS

I would like to express my deepest gratitude to everyone who supported me throughout the journey of creating this book. To my family and friends, your unwavering encouragement and patience have been invaluable.

A special thanks to my team, whose expertise and guidance were crucial in developing the dietary plans and recipes shared in this book. Your insights have been a cornerstone of this work.

I am also deeply grateful to my editor, Michael Jones, for your meticulous attention to detail and for helping shape this book into a comprehensive and accessible guide.

To the support groups and communities who shared their experiences and provided feedback, your contributions have enriched this book and made it more relatable for those living with fructose intolerance.

Lastly, to my readers, thank you for embarking on this journey with me. I hope this book provides you with the knowledge and tools to navigate your dietary needs and improve your quality of life.

COPYRIGHT

Copyright © Chris Preston, RDN. All rights reserved.

No part of this publication may be reproduced, distributed, or transmitted in any form or by any means, including photocopying, recording, or other electronic or mechanical methods, without the prior written permission of the publisher, except in the case of brief quotations embodied in critical reviews and certain other noncommercial uses permitted by copyright law.

This book is intended to provide general information about diet and nutrition. It is not intended as a substitute for professional medical advice, diagnosis, or treatment. Always seek the advice of your physician or other qualified health provider with any questions you may have regarding a medical condition.

TABLE OF CONTENTS

ACKNOWLEDGEMENTS 2

COPYRIGHT 4

TABLE OF CONTENTS 5

UNDERSTANDING VITILIGO AND ITS IMPACT ON DIET 1

    Causes and Risk factors of Vitiligo 9

    Symptoms and Diagnosis 16

    Treatment 20

    Complications of Vitiligo 28

    How Diet Can Influence Vitiligo 33

    Importance of Nutrition in Managing Vitiligo 39

NUTRIENTS AND FOODS BENEFICIAL FOR VITILIGO 42

    Antioxidants and Their Role in Vitiligo Management 47

Vitamins C, E, and B12 for Vitiligo Management 50

Importance of Zinc and Copper 55

Omega-3 Fatty Acids and Their Anti-inflammatory Properties 61

FOODS TO AVOID OR LIMIT FOR VITILIGO . 66

The Role of Gluten and Dairy in Autoimmune Conditions 68

Foods with High Histamine Levels 71

Processed Foods and Their Impact on Skin Health 85

Alcohol and Caffeine: Their Effects on Vitiligo 87

DELICIOUSLY SIMPLE RECIPES YOU MUST TRY! 90

BREAKFAST RECIPES FOR VITILIGO 91

Gluten-free banana pancakes 91

Green goddess smoothie bowl 93

Summer porridge 96

Vegan breakfast muffins 98

Crumpets 100

Raspberry coconut porridge 103

Chocolate crumpets 104

Beetroot pancakes... 107

Berry omelette 109

Creamy smoked haddock & saffron kedgeree
.... 111

Kale & salmon kedgeree 113

Cured salmon 116

Strawberry-Pineapple Smoothie 120

Chickpea & Potato Hash 121

Cheddar and Zucchini Frittata 123

Spinach & Feta Scrambled Egg Pitas 125

Baked Eggs in Tomato Sauce with Kale 126

LUNCH RECIPES FOR VITILIGO 129

Vegetarian lasagne 129

Tomato, watermelon & feta salad with mint dressing 133

Asparagus & lentil salad with cranberries & crumbled feta 134

Roasted summer vegetable casserole 136

Sweet potato jackets with pomegranate & celeriac slaw 138

Bean, tomato & watercress salad 141

Lemon roast vegetables with yogurt tahini & pomegranate 142

BBQ mackerel 144

Korean fishcakes with fried eggs & spicy salsa 146

Classic lasagne 150

Haddock in tomato basil sauce 153

Antipasti salmon 156

Sticky onion & cheddar quiche 159

Steamed bass with pak choi 162

Mackerel with orange & harissa glaze 164

DINNER RECIPES FOR VITILIGO 167

Black bean chilli 167

One-pot chicken & rice 169

Roast chicken with lemon & rosemary roots 171

Lemony chicken stew with giant couscous ... 174

Vegetarian carbonara 177

Healthy fish korma 180

Smoked salmon soufflés 183

Stir-fried chicken with broccoli & brown rice
.... 186

Chicken & chorizo ragu 188

Steaks with goulash sauce & sweet potato fries 190

Minty griddled chicken & peach salad 194

Spinach kedgeree with spiced salmon 197

Mustard salmon & veg bake with horseradish sauce 200

Hake fish cakes with mustard middles 202

Baked sea bream with tomatoes & coriander 207

Herby fish fingers 209

Salmon & lemon mini fish cakes 211

SOUP RECIPES FOR VITILIGO 214

Corn & split pea chowder 214

Broccoli and kale green soup 216

Fresh tomato soup with cheesy cornbread 219

Summer pistou 222

Spinach soup 224

Red lentil soup 227

Courgette, pea & pesto soup 228

Broccoli & stilton soup 230

Chicken & sweetcorn soup 233

Moroccan spiced cauliflower & almond soup 235

Leek, fennel & potato soup with cashel blue cheese 237

Smoky tomato, chipotle & charred corn soup 239

Creamy pumpkin & lentil soup 241

Chorizo & chickpea soup 243

White velvet soup with smoky almonds 245

LIFESTYLE TIPS AND ADDITIONAL CONSIDERATIONS 248

Coping and support..250

PART I
UNDERSTANDING VITILIGO AND ITS IMPACT ON DIET

Vitiligo (vit-ih-LIE-go) is a disease that causes loss of skin color in patches. The discolored areas usually get bigger with time. The condition can affect the skin on any part of the body. It can also affect hair and the inside of the mouth.

Normally, the color of hair and skin is determined by melanin. Vitiligo occurs when cells that produce melanin die or stop functioning. Vitiligo affects people of all skin types, but it may be more noticeable in people with brown or Black skin, because the contrast between normal skin tone and the white patches affected by vitiligo is more pronounced.

The condition is not life-threatening or contagious. It can be stressful or make you feel bad about yourself. People with vitiligo experience skin color loss in various areas of the body. Often it's symmetrical, affecting both sides, such as the left and right hands or both knees. Other vitiligo symptoms include discoloration in the mouth, on the scalp, or of hair, eyelashes, or eyebrows.

Treatment for vitiligo may restore color to the affected skin. But it doesn't prevent continued loss of skin color or a recurrence.

Types of Vitiligo

According to the American Academy of Dermatology, there are multiple types of vitiligo depending on the appearance of the patches, how much of the body they cover, and how they spread.

These types can include:

Localized vitiligo

A doctor may diagnose localized vitiligo if only a few patches cover a small area. These patches may develop in a few places on the body.

Nonsegmental vitiligo

The most common type of vitiligo, with pale skin patches usually appearing on both sides of the body. The first signs may show up on hands, fingertips, wrists, around the eyes or mouth, or on the feet. Nonsegmental vitiligo is also called bilateral or generalized vitiligo or vitiligo vulgaris, according to research.

Nonsegmental vitiligo is divided into subtypes based on the way the condition shows up. These include acrofacial vitiligo, which appears on the face, hands, and feet; mucosal vitiligo, which affects the mucous membranes of the mouth, nose, and genitals; localized or focal vitiligo, which occurs on just a few areas of the body; and universal vitiligo, which may involve 80 to 90 percent of an affected person's skin, according to research.

Nonsegmental vitiligo is the more common type.

Some researchers consider the following types of vitiligo as subtypes of nonsegmental vitiligo:

Acrofacial: This occurs mainly on the face, on the scalp, around the genitals, and on the fingers or toes.

Mucosal: This appears mostly around the mucous membranes and lips.

Generalized: In generalized vitiligo, there is no specific area or size of patches. This type causes scattered patches on different areas of the body.

Universal: In this rare type of vitiligo, depigmentation covers most of the body.

Mixed: This type of vitiligo is also rare. It can cause a person to have both segmental and nonsegmental vitiligo.

Rare variants: This includes other rare variations of vitiligo.

Segmental vitiligo

Segmental vitiligo can cause rapid color loss on one side of the body. For this type, white patches often appear on just one side of the body, such as one arm or one leg instead of both. Loss of hair color is common. Segmental vitiligo can begin early in life. It may spread rapidly for six months to two years, However, after 6–12 months, it can be more constant, stable, and less erratic than the nonsegmental type. Once it stops, many people with segmental vitiligo do not develop new patches.

In rare cases, this form of vitiligo may become active again years later. About 5 to 16 percent of vitiligo cases are segmental vitiligo.

According to a 2020 review article, segmental vitiligo is less common and affects only about 5–16% of people with vitiligo.

Furthermore, it most often appears at a younger age than nonsegmental vitiligo and only affects one body area, such as one leg, one side of the face, or one arm.

Segmental vitiligo:

Conventional vitiligo treatments, such as topical steroids and phototherapy, may not work for this type.

Vitiligo vs. Tinea Versicolor

Tinea versicolor is a fungal skin infection of the skin. Unlike vitiligo, where the milky-white patches are smooth milky white, tinea versicolor causes white, brown, tan, and salmon scaly patches. Tinea versicolor goes away after being treated with antifungal medications you take by mouth or apply on your skin, but it may return. Vitiligo doesn't go away at all.

A doctor may be the best person to tell what condition may be causing your skin symptoms.

Vitiligo vs. Albinism

Albinism is a skin condition that runs in the family. It happens you have inherited mutated genes that cause abnormal melanocytes that can't properly make or distribute melanin throughout the skin, causing your skin, hair, and eyes to look pale.

In vitiligo, on the other hand, melanocytes are destroyed and the affected areas of the skin appear in milky-white patches.

Also, albinism appears at birth, whereas vitiligo usually develops over time and typically appears before age 40.

Studies are ongoing about whether vitiligo can be passed down; they indicate that 30% of vitiligo cases are genetic.

Causes and Risk factors of Vitiligo

What causes vitiligo?

Vitiligo is due to the loss or destruction of melanocytes (melanin-producing cells).

Genetic factors appear to contribute to 80% of vitiligo risk, whilst environmental factors account for 20%. Many genetic loci have been identified, all related to the immune system, except for TYR which encodes tyrosinase, a key enzyme in melanin production and a major autoantigen in vitiligo.

The convergence or integrated theory combines immunological, biochemical, oxidative, and environmental mechanisms that work jointly in those with a genetic susceptibility is widely accepted.

This could be explained through three phases:

- **Initial phase:** less adhesive melanocytes are prone to internal and external oxidative stresses, leading to the production of more toxic reactive oxygen species (ROS).

- **Progression phase:** an imbalance between ROS and antioxidants will activate the adaptive immune system bridged by the innate immune system.

CD8+ cytotoxic cells release cytokines, mainly interferon-γ (INF-γ) that activate the JAK-STAT pathway through its receptors on keratinocytes.

This will lead to the production of chemokines (CXC), predominantly by keratinocytes, but also by melanocytes themselves, leading to IFN-γ- CXCR3- CXCL9/10 axis loop feedback.

Acting together on their common CXCR3 receptor, CXCL9 drives the main bulk of CD8+ cell homing, while CXCL10 promotes their localisation to affected skin lesions and induction of melanocyte apoptosis through CXC3B activation. Of note, where both humoral (antibody) and T-cell responses appear to be implicated, antibody titres do not correlate with disease activity nor the localisation of distinct vitiligo lesions.

- **Maintenance phase:** established lesions are maintained by resident melanocyte reactive T-cells (TRM cells), through the IL15-dependent pathway. These TRM cells may be responsible for what is called an 'autoimmune memory', in which relapses occur mostly at the same exact site of previous lesions.

Understanding the molecular pathogenesis of vitiligo serves as a promising source for the development of more targeted therapies.

Risk Factors

Vitiligo affects 0.5-2% of the population.

- **Race:** relatively consistent incidence in all races, but appears to be:
    - Less common in the Han Chinese population
    - More common in India (up to 8.8% of the population).

- **Sex:** both men and women appear to be equally affected

Women tend to constitute a higher percentage of overall outpatient visits, due to greater concerns about cosmetic appearance.

- **Onset:** the average age of onset is between 20–24 years, but can occur at any age. Typically, there are two peaks of onset, early (<10 years) or late (around 30 years).

  o 41% of segmental vitiligo cases start before the age of 10.
  o 50% of non-segmental vitiligo cases start before the age of 20.
  o 80% of all cases present before the age of 30.

- **Family History and Genes**: About 20 percent of people with vitiligo have at least one close relative affected by this skin disorder, and researchers have found that having a certain genetic profile makes people more susceptible to developing vitiligo. Variations in over 30 genes have been identified that are associated with vitiligo, including two called NLRP1 and PTPN22. These and other genes now linked with vitiligo are known to be involved with immune-system regulation and inflammation.

• **Environmental Triggers:** Vitiligo seems to be the result of both a preexisting genetic makeup and something in the environment setting off an autoimmune response that destroys melanocytes. Potential triggers include sunburn, exposure to certain chemicals, and trauma or injury to the skin. These triggers can also prompt vitiligo to spread in people who already have the condition.

Autoimmune disease development has been associated with generalized vitiligo, the most common type of vitiligo, especially if there is a family history of vitiligo and other autoimmune disorders.

- The strongest association is with thyroid disease, which can affect up to 15% of adults and 5–10% of children with vitiligo.

- Other less frequently associated autoimmune disorders with vitiligo are:

    o Rheumatoid arthritis
    o Insulin-dependent diabetes mellitus (mostly adult-onset)
    o Pernicious anaemia (B12 deficiency)
    o Addison disease
    o Systemic lupus erythematosus
    o Alopecia areata
    o Other autoimmune dermatologic conditions, eg, psoriasis and lichen sclerosus.

Vitiligo is also three times more common in recipients of allogeneic bone marrow and stem-cell transplants than in the healthy population.

Symptoms and Diagnosis

Symptoms

You'll often lose pigment quickly on several areas of your skin. After the white patches appear, they may stay the same for a while but get bigger later. You may have cycles of pigment loss and stability.

Vitiligo commonly affects:

- Body folds (such as armpits)
- Places that have been injured in the past
- Areas exposed to the sun
- Around moles

- Around body openings
- Mucous membranes (tissues that line your nose and mouth)
- Eyelids
- Hair

It's rare for pigment to return once the white patches have developed.

You may also have symptoms of other autoimmune diseases along with vitiligo, such as:

- A goiter or enlarged thyroid glands
- Anemia or low levels of healthy red blood cells
- Extreme weight and muscle loss
- Premature grey hair
- Patchy hair loss
- Weakness

Diagnosis

If you suspect you may have vitiligo, visit your primary care doctor or a dermatologist. To evaluate a vitiligo diagnosis, your doctor will likely ask about risk factors such as:

Whether a close relative has been diagnosed with vitiligo

Whether you have been diagnosed with an autoimmune disorder

If you've experienced recent stress (such as a major life change) or other potentially triggering events (such as a severe sunburn)

Most of the time, doctors diagnose vitiligo by visually examining white patches on the skin and considering your medical history. Your physician may use a Wood's lamp, which uses ultraviolet light to identify pigment loss. This lamp is especially useful for people with fairer skin, where the difference in skin color can be subtler.

Some dermatologists will want to do more testing beyond a skin exam. Your doctor may order a skin biopsy, which will show whether melanocytes are present in the skin. A lack of melanocytes is an indication of vitiligo. Your doctor may also ask for a blood test to see if you have another autoimmune disease.

Additionally, they may also perform an eye exam for uveitis, a form of eye inflammation that can be associated with vitiligo. Your doctor will also rule out other skin conditions that can look similar to vitiligo, such as skin damage from exposure to industrial chemicals called chemical leukoderma; tinea versicolor, a yeast infection that can lighten or darken areas of skin; and albinism, a genetic condition marked by low levels of melanin in skin, hair, and eyes.

Treatment

The American Academy of Dermatology describes vitiligo as "more than a cosmetic problem." It is a health issue that needs medical attention.

Several remedies can help decrease the visibility of the condition, though some people may not want to treat the condition at all.

Using sunscreen

The American Academy of Dermatology recommends using sunscreen to protect the skin. The lighter patches of skin are especially sensitive to sunlight, and they can burn quickly. A dermatologist can advise on a suitable type of sunscreen.

Phototherapy with UVB light

A common treatment option is exposure to certain wavelengths of ultraviolet B (UVB) light, called phototherapy. Home phototherapy units are available but must be used with the supervision of a physician.

If a person goes to a clinic for treatment, a healthcare professional may recommend two to three visits per week.

If there are white spots across large body areas, UVB phototherapy may help. It involves full-body treatment in an office setting.

UVB phototherapy, combined with other treatments, can positively affect vitiligo. However, the result is not predictable, and there is still no treatment to fully re-pigment the skin.

Phototherapy with UVA light

Done in a healthcare setting, UVA treatment involves people taking a drug that increases their skin's sensitivity to UV light. Then, in a series of treatments, a qualified healthcare professional exposes the affected skin to prescribed doses of UVA light.

According to a 2017 meta-analysis, progress is typically evident after 6–12 months of therapy.

Skin camouflage

While many people feel comfortable or enjoy how vitiligo looks, it may not be comfortable for everyone with the condition.

In cases of mild vitiligo, a person can camouflage the white patches with colored cosmetic creams and makeup. They can select tones that best match their skin tone.

Topical corticosteroids

Corticosteroid ointments are creams containing steroids. A 2017 review of studies concludes that applying topical corticosteroids to the white patches is an effective treatment.

Corticosteroids should be used with caution on the face and only under the guidance of a physician because of potential side effects, such as:

• thinning of the skin

• Spider veins

• Acne lesions

Calcipotriene (Dovonex)

Calcipotriene is a form of vitamin D used in topical therapy, often in combination with corticosteroids or phototherapy. Side effects may include:

- itching

- Redness

- burning

Drugs affecting the immune system

The topical medications tacrolimus and pimecrolimus are drugs known as calcineurin inhibitors. They may help with smaller patches of depigmentation.

However, pimecrolimus contains a boxed warning from the Food and Drug Administration (FDA) about rare cases of malignancy, such as skin cancer and lymphoma, reported in people treated with calcineurin inhibitors.

Skin grafts

In a skin graft, a surgeon carefully removes healthy patches of pigmented skin and uses them to cover affected areas.

This procedure is not very common because it takes time and can result in scarring in the area.

Blister grafting involves producing a blister on more typical skin using suction. The top of the blister is then removed and placed on an area where the pigment was lost.

Tattooing

Micropigmentation, or medical tattooing, includes implanting pigment into the skin. It may work in people with light to medium skin tones.

Drawbacks can include difficulty matching the color of skin and the fact that tattoos fade but do not tan. Sometimes, skin damage caused by tattooing can trigger another patch of vitiligo.

Depigmentation

Depigmentation can be an option when the affected area is widespread, covering half of the body or more. It works by reducing the skin color in unaffected parts to match the whiter areas better.

Depigmentation involves applying strong topical lotions or ointments, such as monobenzyl ether of hydroquinone (MBEH), 4-methoxyphenol, and phenol.

The treatment is permanent, but it can make the skin more fragile. In addition, people must avoid extended exposure to the sun. Depigmentation can take 1–4 years depending on the depth of the original skin tone.

Ruxolitinib (Opzelura)

Opzelura is a topical Janus kinase (JAK) inhibitor. It's the only medication approved by the FDA to restore lost pigment in people with vitiligo. It can treat a small area of the body in people 12 years and older with nonsegmental vitiligo.

Prevention of Vitiligo

There's currently no way to prevent the onset of vitiligo, but there are steps you can take that may help keep vitiligo symptoms from worsening. In addition to the treatment options mentioned above, protect your skin from the sun and UV light by using sunscreen, seeking shade, and wearing clothing that protects you from harmful rays. Cuts, scrapes, burns, and tattoos can trigger patches of vitiligo in some people. In general, try to avoid injuring your skin.

Complications of Vitiligo

In general, people who have been diagnosed with vitiligo do not need to be overly worried about developing serious complications.

Vitiligo and Skin Cancer Risk

People with vitiligo — like the rest of the population — are encouraged to wear sunscreen (specifically a broad-spectrum, water-resistant option with an SPF of 30 or higher.

Part of that is because skin without its natural color is more likely to burn in the sun. A function of melanin (the pigment that gives skin color, which is missing in patches of skin in people with vitiligo) is to help block out some of the sun's dangerous ultraviolet rays, so skin without it may be more vulnerable to sun damage.

But sun protection is also important because avoiding getting tan can make vitiligo patches less noticeable, and some vitiligo treatments can be disrupted by sun exposure.

Since the skin in the vitiligo-affected areas can burn more easily, it may be surprising to learn that instead of increasing skin cancer risk, vitiligo is associated with lower risk. One study found a threefold lower risk for melanoma and nonmelanoma skin cancers in people with vitiligo compared with those without it.

There are a few theories for why this might happen. The same genes associated with vitiligo may also lower the risk of malignant melanoma, suggested one study.

A second theory posits that whatever's causing the immune system to destroy melanocytes also causes it to destroy cancerous cells.

It's good news for people with vitiligo, but it doesn't mean they should rely on their condition to give them absolute protection against the effects of the sun. Those with vitiligo simply don't need to be any more worried about skin cancer than the rest of the population.

Vitiligo and Other Autoimmune Disorders

Up to one-quarter of patients with vitiligo have another autoimmune disease. If you have vitiligo, you may be at risk for an autoimmune disorder. So it's important to discuss any new or unusual health issues you're experiencing with your primary care practitioner. Vitiligo does not cause other autoimmune conditions, but it may share a genetic basis with one.

Here are some of the most common autoimmune diseases associated with vitiligo:

- Autoimmune thyroid disease

- Rheumatoid arthritis

- Type 1 diabetes

- Psoriasis

- Pernicious anemia

- Addison's disease

- Systemic lupus erythematosus

Vitiligo and Mental Health Complications

A big concern when it comes to vitiligo complications is the emotional toll of living with a very visible skin condition, especially one that can begin early in life.

It can be especially difficult for people with darker skin, because the differences in skin tone are more obvious. For people with light skin, the presence of vitiligo may be less noticeable.

And for children and teens, it may be challenging to cope with vitiligo in the midst of other changes happening to their bodies, minds, and emotions — especially if their peers don't understand or respond sensitively to what's happening. For many, learning to deal with vitiligo means finding someone to talk to about the experience, whether that's a trusted doctor, close family members or friends, or a mental health professional.

How Diet Can Influence Vitiligo

There is so far no evidence that confirms a direct link between nutrition and vitiligo. However, some studies suggest changing your diet or adding supplements could have a positive impact.

A nutrient-dense diet is always advisable, not only for vitiligo but for optimum health. A plant-based diet rich in antioxidants, low in inflammatory foods and possibly also gluten-free, may have a beneficial effect on vitiligo.

Here are some management tips for improving your vitiligo symptoms with a change in diet and nutrition:

1. Eat an antioxidant-rich diet to help improve your vitiligo symptoms.

One potential cause of vitiligo is the effect of stress on the cells that produce melanin — less melanin means more skin depigmentation.

You can try to protect yourself against this stress by eating a diet high in antioxidants. One study carried out on mice with vitiligo showed significant levels of repigmentation when they ate foods high in antioxidants.

Vegetables, fruits, nuts, seeds and spices are all high in antioxidants. A good rule of thumb for eating enough antioxidants is to eat as many different coloured fruits and vegetables as possible: "eat the rainbow".

Foods high in omega-3 (but lower in omega-6) could also help improve your symptoms. These include oily fish, nuts, seeds and algae.

A plant-based diet has been shown to be very high in antioxidants (as well as a whole host of other benefits!). This is not the same as a vegan diet because you can still eat some animal products. However, the majority of your diet is made up of plants.

2. Try a gluten-free diet for vitiligo.

One study on a vitiligo patient found that following a gluten-free diet resulted in substantial repigmentation. The case study saw significant changes after a nine-month period.

The study was only carried out on one person, but you could cut gluten from your diet to see if it works for you.

One reason for the improvements in this patient could be because gluten is an inflammatory food.

3. Avoid inflammatory foods for vitiligo.

Avoiding foods that cause an inflammatory response may help reduce the symptoms of vitiligo.

Inflammatory foods include:

- Processed meats

- Sugary drinks

- Trans fats, found in fried foods

- White bread

- White pasta

- Gluten

- Soybean oil and vegetable oil

- Processed snack foods, such as chips and crackers

- Desserts, such as cookies, candy, and ice cream

- Excess alcohol

- Excessive carbohydrates

Inflammatory foods make it harder for your gut to work and remain healthy. A healthy gut helps decrease low-grade inflammation in the body. Fibre, probiotic and prebiotic foods, such as sauerkraut, can help improve gut health.

4. Take supplements for vitiligo.

Although it is considered preferable to consume nutrients via whole foods rather than with supplements, studies suggest some supplements can aid repigmentation in vitiligo patients:

- Ginkgo biloba

- Alpha lipoic acid

- Vitamin C

- Vitamin E

- Polyunsaturated fatty acids (omega-3)

- Vitamin D

Is there any link between vitiligo and food allergies?

As far as we are aware there is no research to show that vitiligo can either be caused from food allergies, or that you are more likely to have such allergies if you have vitiligo.

Importance of Nutrition in Managing Vitiligo

Nutrition plays a vital role in managing vitiligo, a condition characterized by skin pigment loss. While it can't cure vitiligo on its own, nutrition significantly impacts its progression and overall skin health. Here's why nutrition matters:

1. Antioxidant Protection: Vitiligo is linked to oxidative stress, where free radicals harm melanocytes (cells producing pigment). Antioxidants like vitamins C and E, found in fruits, veggies, and nuts, help counteract these free radicals and protect melanocytes.

2. Balanced Micronutrients: Adequate intake of zinc, copper, vitamin B12, and folic acid supports healthy skin and melanin production. Deficiencies in these nutrients can hinder melanocyte function and worsen vitiligo.

3. Supports Immune System: Some evidence suggests autoimmune factors contribute to vitiligo. Nutrients like vitamin D and omega-3 fatty acids help regulate immune responses and reduce inflammation, potentially slowing down autoimmune processes.

4. Gut Health Importance: Emerging research links gut health to autoimmune conditions like vitiligo. A diet rich in fiber, probiotics (yogurt, fermented foods), and prebiotics (fruits, veggies, whole grains) supports a healthy gut microbiome, which may benefit immune function and skin health.

5. Avoiding Trigger Foods: While specific foods' role in vitiligo is unclear, some report certain foods or additives worsen symptoms. Tracking diet can help identify potential triggers.

6. Enhances Skin Health: Nutrition supports overall skin health crucial for those with vitiligo. Hydrating foods like cucumbers, watermelon, and oranges maintain skin hydration, while omega-3-rich foods (salmon, nuts) support skin integrity.

7. Mental Well-being: Vitiligo impacts mental health. A balanced diet promotes overall well-being and a positive mindset.

PART II

NUTRIENTS AND FOODS BENEFICIAL FOR VITILIGO

Some experts suggest following a plant-based diet because it's rich in antioxidants.

While a plant-based diet can provide general health benefits, there's no strong evidence behind this diet to directly benefit a person with vitiligo.

Instead, focus on a balanced diet that includes antioxidant-rich fruits and vegetables, whole grains, lean proteins, and healthy fat to support a healthy immune system. Options include:

- **Fruits and vegetables:** Focus on eating antioxidant-rich fruits and vegetables. Choose non-starchy vegetables like broccoli, asparagus, Brussels sprouts, beets, carrots, cauliflower, green beans, and spinach. Eat more fruits like berries, oranges, melon, and apples. (Deeper, darker-colored fruits and vegetables usually contain more antioxidants.)

- **Whole grains:** Try to limit or avoid refined grains as these are usually stripped of key nutrients found in whole grains. Consume grains and foods like brown rice, whole-wheat pasta, oats, and quinoa.

- **Protein:** The best protein sources are lean cuts of meat, including skinless chicken and turkey, eggs, and legumes such as lentils, peas, and beans. Fatty fish like salmon and tuna are great sources of omega-3 fatty acids that work to protect your heart and lower inflammation. Limit processed meat like hot dogs, salami, and lunch meat. Try to limit your red meat consumption to no more than twice per week and try to include more plant-based protein like legumes.

- **Processed foods:** Eating too many processed foods can cause inflammation and usually have little to no nutritional value. Focus on enjoying desserts, sugary beverages, and pre-packaged foods in small quantities.

- **Beverages:** The best beverage to drink is plain water. If you choose to drink other beverages, avoid alcohol and those with added sugars like juice, sports drinks, and soda. Opt for unsweet tea, seltzer water, and coffee without sugar.

- **Healthy fats**: It's important to get enough healthy fats in as part of a balanced diet. Foods like avocado, chia seeds, and nut butter are all great sources of healthy fat.

Dietary supplements

According to a 2021 review, some research suggests that taking one or more of the following supplements may help improve symptoms of vitiligo:

- vitamin B12 and folic acid
- vitamin D
- vitamin E

Some studies have also found potential benefits from taking certain herbal supplements, such as ginkgo biloba and a component in green tea called epigallocatechin-3-gallate.

However, the research evidence is limited, and not all studies have found benefits from taking supplements for vitiligo. More research is necessary to learn whether certain supplements can help treat this condition.

A person should speak with a doctor before taking a dietary or herbal supplement. The doctor can help them understand the potential benefits and risks.

In some cases, a doctor may order blood tests to determine whether the individual has low levels of certain nutrients. A doctor may also refer someone with vitiligo to a dietitian, who can help devise a suitable eating plan.

Antioxidants and Their Role in Vitiligo Management

The Potential of Antioxidants

A systematic review of 14 studies from 2003 to 2023 explored the link between diet and vitiligo. The review noted the anti-inflammatory properties of Vitamins C, D, and B12 and their role in reducing reactive oxygen species (ROS), which can aid in managing vitiligo. Combining these vitamins with topical corticosteroids has shown effectiveness, although hyper-doses of Vitamin C may actually worsen the condition. Vitamin D's role remains controversial; a small and controversial study suggests that high-dose, short-term supplementation can improve repigmentation, though a standard dose of up to 4,000 IU daily is generally beneficial. Polyunsaturated fatty acids (PUFAs) and Alpha

Lipoic Acid (ALA) are thought to modulate the immune system beneficially, yet despite their antioxidant properties, they did not significantly improve outcomes.

Genetic Analysis and Antioxidant Therapy

Another groundbreaking study from China evaluated the effects of antioxidant dietary supplements and diet-derived circulating antioxidants on vitiligo using MR analysis. It found that coffee, red wine, and standard tea — all rich in antioxidants — acted as protective factors against vitiligo. These beverages help clear free radicals, enhance plasma reductase activity, and balance the accumulation of ROS.

Coffee, in particular, is a robust source of dietary antioxidants, containing various phytochemicals that scavenge free radicals and modulate the immune response. Red wine, rich in phenols, enhances the serum's antioxidant capacity and protects against peroxidation-induced damage. Tea, with its high content of polyphenols, offers significant antioxidant activity that varies with its cultivation and processing.

Clinical Guidelines and Future Directions

The European Dermatology Forum Consensus suggests that combining phototherapy with oral antioxidants might enhance treatment outcomes, particularly by counteracting the oxidative stress induced by UV radiation. While promising, these findings, mostly based on a European population, may not be universally applicable.

Vitamins C, E, and B12 for Vitiligo Management

For years, scientists have been trying to find a connection between diet and vitiligo. Although no one particular nutrient has been identified as a 'cure', it is evident that Vitamin B12 – Folic Acid, Vitamin C, antioxidants including vitamins A and E, beta carotene and minerals such as selenium, copper, and zinc are involved in pigmentation and maintaining healthy skin.

Vitamin A, C, and E

These vitamins act as antioxidants and prevent epidermal oxidative stress, which is considered as a contributory factor for the premature destruction of melanocytes.

Vitamin C (found in vegetables and citrus fruits) is particularly needed for the enzymes which are involved in skin pigmentation. Being an antioxidant, Vitamin C helps to maintain the body's immune system.

Vitamin B12

Vitamin B12 promotes healthy hair, skin, and nails. It helps to regulate the production of pigment in the skin. Keeping such a hypothesis in mind, many researchers have attempted to evaluate the role of vitamin B12 in the development of vitiligo.

Experts believe if approached correctly, vitamin B12 can potentially prevent the death of melanocytes, thus preventing the loss of pigment in vitiligo. In many studies, Vitamin B12 and folic acid levels are decreased in vitiligo patients –

important cofactors for the metabolism of homocysteine. Therefore, it is possible that increased homocysteine plays a role in the destruction of melanocytes.

Vitamin B12 deficiency can be tamed by supplementation under the guidance of a licensed medical professional. It should be ideally balanced with other water-soluble vitamins. Vitamin B12 is only found in animal products. Some grains and plant-based milk are also fortified with vitamin B12.

Vitamin D

Past pieces of evidence support strong links between vitamin D deficiency and autoimmune conditions. Since the vitamin helps in maintaining the immune system, a vitamin D deficiency has been observed in many autoimmune disorders.

Keeping such a hypothesis in mind, many researchers have been evaluating the role of vitamin D status in vitiligo as well.

Vitamin D is synthesized in the skin. As revealed in studies, it increases the rate of melanogenesis by increasing the activity of tyrosinase. It protects the epidermal melanin unit and restores melanocyte by controlling the activation, proliferation, and migration of melanocytes. This makes researchers anticipate that vitamin D could be a potent immunomodulator.

Vitamin D deficiency could be controlled by supplementation under the supervision of a licensed medical physician. It should be balanced with other fat-soluble vitamins. Vitamin D2 is present in fungi/yeast while cholecalciferol vitamin D 3 is found in foods of animal origin (such as fatty fish). Other sources include eggs, milk, cheese, and cereals.

Folic Acid

Vitamin B12 inhibits the production of homocysteine, which downregulates the activity of tyrosinase (an enzyme responsible for melanin production). In this whole process, folic acid works alongside vitamin B12 as a methyl group donor. Hence, a combination of vitamin B12 and folic acid supplementation in addition to sun exposure is a good strategy to regain natural skin color in vitiligo. Folic acid is mostly found in green leafy vegetables, yeast extract, offal, and wholegrain cereals. In some countries, it is also added to breakfast cereals and bread.

Beta carotene

An antioxidant and a precursor form of vitamin A, Beta carotene can be found in all dark green, orange and yellow vegetables and fruits. It plays an important role in maintaining normal skin color. It is also responsible for skin deposition of dietary carotenoids (any of a class of mainly yellow, orange, or red fat-soluble pigments). It provides photoprotection for lightly pigmented skins. Carrot is one good source of Beta carotene.

Importance of Zinc and Copper

Many sources can be sited to confirm that certain metal ions including zinc (Zn) and copper are found in high levels in pigmented tissues that are involved in melanin synthesis. This only illustrates zinc's far-reaching effects in vitiligo's better management. Keeping in mind that zinc stimulates the melanocytes into action and increases melanin and repigmentation in the skin, scientists across the world have attempted to evaluate the role of zinc status in the prevention and treatment of vitiligo.

Signs of zinc deficiency in individuals with vitiligo

Estimates hint that about 25% of the world's population (every fourth individual in the world) is at risk of zinc deficiency. You too might have a zinc deficiency along with vitiligo if you:

Have alcohol addiction.

Are diagnosed with chronic diarrhea, chronic kidney disease, chronic liver disease, diabetes, pancreatic disease or ulcerative colitis.

May not have access to a variety of foods.

Eat higher volumes of legumes, nuts, beans, soybeans, and whole-grain foods.

At times, zinc deficiency can be caused by a diet high in processed foods and foods grown in zinc-deficient soil. Zinc and Copper have a very close relationship. When properly balanced (best in the range of 8:1 to 12:1 zinc to copper ratio), they work synergistically. Factors such as stress or diet can reduce zinc levels, causing an increase in copper, creating an unhealthy imbalance over time.

How is zinc deficiency related to vitiligo?

Several studies have shown that people with vitiligo are often deficient in certain vitamins (D, B12) folic acid, and minerals like zinc and copper. Since nutritional deficiencies are known to alter melanin production, melanocyte degeneration is found greater in active vitiligo. Additionally, Zinc deficiencies have been reported to induce hypopigmentation (characterized specifically as an area of skin becoming lighter than the baseline skin color) in various animals.

A study included 50 participants with vitiligo and 50 apparently healthy controls. Serum Zinc (Zn) levels were measured in each study group. Serum Zn levels were found statistically significantly lower in both the studied groups but were much lower in the vitiligo group than the control group.

Over the years, researchers have suggested that vitiligo could be a result of autoimmunity, oxidative stress or neural causes. However, the exact cause and subsequent development of vitiligo have not been fully understood. But, it has been established that zinc is another cofactor in melanin production, and many people with vitiligo are found low in zinc levels. Hence, it is worth checking if supplementing with the mineral can help the skin disorder to slow down.

Treatment of zinc deficiency in people with vitiligo

If people with vitiligo are deficient in zinc, then its supplementation and dietary changes can help them manage the progression of the white patches. Since many research studies focused on zinc's role in pigmentation are underway, it's recommended to go for zinc supplementation under the guidance of a licensed healthcare professional. Being, a trace element, zinc is required in minutely small doses. Hence always seek advice from your doctor for the suitable dosages.

Conventionally used for skin health, Aloe Vera supports proper nutrient absorption and contains essential minerals like zinc. One can alternatively increase their intake of zinc-containing foods such as oysters, fortified breakfast cereals, baked beans, milk, yogurt, beef chuck roast, chickpeas, and plain oatmeal.

Zinc and Copper are interrelated. When properly balanced (8:1 to 12:1 zinc to copper ratio), they work synergistically. Factors such as stress or an unhealthy diet can reduce zinc levels, causing an increase in copper and resulting in nutritional imbalance.

Conventionally used for skin health, Aloe Vera contains essential minerals like zinc and copper. One can alternatively increase their intake of oysters, fortified breakfast cereals, baked beans, milk, yogurt, beef chuck roast, chickpeas, and plain oatmeal to overcome zinc insufficiency. Apart from supplementation, drinking water out of copper vessels can also be beneficial for copper deficiency in vitiligo.

Omega-3 Fatty Acids and Their Anti-inflammatory Properties

Studies have shown that increasing the levels of omega-3s in our cell membranes may protect against or help to reduce the symptoms of certain diseases. For example, scientists have discovered that increasing the Omega-3 Index can decrease the risk of death in patients with heart disease and can decrease swollen joints in patients with rheumatoid arthritis. One thing that these ailments have in common is inflammation, which can be reduced by omega-3s.

In many cases, inflammation is a very good thing. It is the process that occurs when the immune system fights back against an infection. Have you ever gotten a splinter, and noticed that the area is swollen, redder than the rest of your skin, and maybe a bit painful? This is inflammation! Your immune system is working hard to fight off any bacteria that may have entered your body when you got the splinter. Normally, once your immune system has eliminated the threat of an infection, the area will heal and return to normal. Unfortunately, sometimes this process goes haywire and inflammation can continue when it is not necessary. This is referred to as chronic inflammation, and it can have many negative effects, including permanent damage to the tissue. Medical concerns including heart disease, arthritis, and even some cancers are associated with chronic inflammation, which is why it is so important to keep inflammation from getting out of control.

Scientists have shown that a high Omega-3 Index can help protect against chronic or uncontrolled inflammation. Specifically, maintaining a proper balance of omega-3s and omega-6s in the diet is critical for maintaining healthy omega-3 levels in the cell membranes. It is important to remember that nutrition is all about balance: we don't want to consume only omega-3s, but instead we should try to eat a healthy proportion of both omega-3s and omega-6s. Scientists recommend that we eat only about 2 times more omega-6s than omega-3s, but it is estimated that most Americans consume more than 20 times more omega-6s than omega-3s! This imbalance in dietary fatty acids may contribute to the chronic inflammatory diseases prevalent in individuals consuming a Western-style diet.

How do omega-3s help reduce inflammation?

This is a question that scientists are still trying to understand, but there are a few discoveries that could explain this. First, having more omega-3s in their cell membranes allows cells to make more omega-3-derived metabolites, many of which can turn off the inflammatory response and turn on a healing response that helps the tissue or cell repair any damage caused by inflammation. Another way omega-3s reduce inflammation could be through changes in types and amounts of microorganisms that live in the gut, called the gut microbiota. It is well known that what we choose to eat influences the microorganisms that live in the gut and that these organisms can influence our health. Scientists have found that consuming omega-3 fatty acids changes the types of microbes in the gut, but it is not yet known exactly how these changes to the microbiota influence inflammation.

These are just two of many potential ways that omega-3s can protect against inflammation.

PART III
FOODS TO AVOID OR LIMIT FOR VITILIGO

Some foods may increase inflammation in the body. These include:

• Processed meat, such as hot dogs and deli meats

• Refined grains, such as white bread, white rice, white pasta, and pastries

• fried foods, such as french fries and chips

• Sugar-sweetened beverages, such as soda

• Desserts, such as cookies, candy, and ice cream

• Excess alcohol

- Excess carbohydrates

Limiting or avoiding these foods may help limit inflammation.

It is also best to avoid foods that contain trans fats. In 2018, the Food and Drug Administration (FDA) banned trans fats in the United States. However, manufacturers in many other countries still add trans fats to processed foods, such as commercial baked goods, margarine, and shortening.

Some people with vitiligo may have gluten sensitivity or intolerance. They may benefit from avoiding gluten, which is present in:

- Wheat and wheat-based flour, including all-purpose flour

- Ancient forms of wheat, including einkorn, emmer, spelt, and khorasan (kamut)

- Barley and barley-based malt

- Rye

A person should speak with a doctor before cutting gluten from their diet. The doctor can help them understand the potential benefits and risks of a gluten-free diet.

The Role of Gluten and Dairy in Autoimmune Conditions

The role of gluten and dairy in vitiligo, a condition marked by skin pigment loss, isn't as extensively researched as in other autoimmune diseases. Here's what we currently know based on available studies and clinical observations:

1. Gluten:

- Celiac Disease Connection: Vitiligo isn't directly linked to celiac disease, which is triggered by gluten in genetically predisposed individuals and affects the gut.

- Non-Celiac Gluten Sensitivity: While gluten sensitivity can cause symptoms in those without celiac disease, its connection to vitiligo isn't well-established.

2. Dairy:

- Autoimmune Considerations: Dairy proteins like casein and whey can potentially trigger immune responses, but evidence linking dairy to vitiligo is inconclusive.

- Mixed Findings: Some reports suggest cutting out dairy may improve vitiligo symptoms for some, but scientific backing is limited.

3. General Dietary Advice:

- Focus on Antioxidants and Nutrients: Eating foods rich in antioxidants (like vitamins C, E, and beta-carotene) and essential nutrients (such as zinc, copper, and vitamin B12) supports skin health and melanocyte function.

- Overall Health Impact: A well-balanced diet that supports overall health and immune function is crucial. This includes staying hydrated and being mindful of potential food triggers based on personal sensitivities.

4. Personalized Approach:

- Consult Healthcare Providers: People with vitiligo should collaborate with healthcare professionals, like dermatologists and dietitians, to determine if dietary adjustments, like eliminating gluten or dairy, might be beneficial.

- Monitoring and Adjustments: Any dietary changes should be carefully monitored to ensure they meet nutritional needs and don't unintentionally affect health negatively.

In essence, while gluten and dairy may influence autoimmune conditions in some instances, their specific impact on vitiligo remains unclear and likely varies among individuals. More research is needed to clarify any connections and to guide personalized dietary recommendations for those managing vitiligo.

Foods with High Histamine Levels

Histamine is a natural chemical that helps your cells communicate. It plays a few important roles in your body, including managing your sleep cycle and supporting your brain function. But it is best known for its role in allergies.

Allergies happen when your immune system overreacts to things such as pollen and mold. Your immune system might mistakenly think that these things, which are usually harmless, could be threats to your body. To defend against the so-called threats, your mast cells (a type of white blood cell) release histamine. The histamine tells your body to launch an allergic reaction.

Seasonal allergies are often the cause of histamine production in the body, but foods can also contain this chemical.

Histamine Intolerance

Most people can tolerate foods high in histamines, but approximately 1% of the population has a histamine intolerance. It tends to be more common in middle age. When you have this condition, you can't break down histamine correctly, causing it to build up in your body. Although it can lead to allergy-like symptoms, it's not considered a food allergy.

It's not clear why some people develop histamine intolerance. Some medications and gut conditions can make it harder for your body to break down histamines. Or you might not have enough diamine oxidase (DAO), the protein that is mainly responsible for breaking down histamine. Low levels of DAO can be caused by genetics (meaning it's passed down through your family), kidney disease, or liver disease.

Histamine intolerance symptoms

Too much histamine triggers an immune response. This can cause symptoms such as:

- Runny or stuffy nose

- Shortness of breath

- Swollen lips, tongue, or throat

- Headaches or migraines

- Fatigue

- Diarrhea

- Bloating

- Nausea or vomiting

- Flushing (redness in the face)

- Itching, rash, or hives

- Irregular or fast heart rate

- Low blood pressure

- Irregular or painful periods

High-Histamine Foods

High histamine foods are often those that are aged, fermented, or soured. They include dairy products, specific fruits and vegetables, processed meats, and alcohol.

Fermented Food

Fermented foods are foods made through the action of bacteria, yeast, fungi, and their enzymes, which oxidize carbohydrates and release energy. These microorganisms may be naturally present in foods.

Fermentation requires the correct amount of microorganisms, proper temperature, pH level (the balance of acid and alkaline), and moisture content.

Examples of fermented foods include:

- Kefir

- Yogurt

- Kombucha

- Kimchi

- Sauerkraut

- Tempe

- Miso

- Sourdough bread

Alcohol

Alcohol is a high-histamine beverage. While some alcohols are a bigger culprit than others (red wine, for example), some people who are concerned about histamine ingestion will avoid all of them.

Examples of high-histamine alcoholic beverages include:

- Wine

- Beer

- Hard cider

- Brown liquors, such as scotch and whiskey

Processed Meat

Processed meats are those that have been salted, fermented, cured, smoked, or otherwise processed to improve the length of preservation. These kinds of meats are high in histamines.

Examples of processed meat include:

- Hot dogs

- Ham

- Sausages

- Beef jerky

- Canned meat

Aged Cheeses

Research has found that certain factors can influence the amount of histamine in cheese, including:

- Bacterial starter culture

- pH level

- Salt level

- Storage temperature

- Ripening time

Aged cheeses have the highest levels of histamine. That's because, during the aging process, proteins break down into histamine. These cheeses include:

- Hard cheese like parmesan, cheddar, romano

- Blue cheeses aged with bacteria, like gorgonzola

- "Stinky" cheeses ripened with bacteria, like Limburger

Dried Fruit

While dried fruits are packed with nutrients, they are also high in histamine. Common dried fruits include:

- Raisins

- Cherries

- Mangoes

- Apricots

- Pineapple

- Apples

- Bananas

Eggplant

Eggplant is a nightshade food that is high in histamine.

Avocado

Avocadoes are high in healthy fats, but they are also high in histamines.

Legumes

Legumes are different than tree nuts. Instead of growing from trees, they grow in pods as edible seeds. Some, but not all, are high in histamines, including:

- Peanuts

- Soybeans

- Peas

- Kidney beans

- Chickpeas

- Green beans

Citrus Fruit

Citrus fruits are those that include citric acid. While not necessarily high in histamine, they may trigger the production of histamines in your body.

Citrus fruits include:

- Oranges

- Lemons

- Limes

Spoiled Fish

Histamine toxicity is a form of food poisoning called scombroid poisoning that occurs from eating spoiled fish. Some fish like mackerel and tuna have high levels of the amino acid histidine, which bacteria can convert to histamine.

Fish that are more prone to causing histamine toxicity, include:

- Tuna

- Mackerel

- Mahi-mahi

- Anchovy

- Herring

- Bluefish

- Amberjack

- Marlin

Low-Histamine Diet

If you are sensitive to high-histamine foods, you may choose to follow a low-histamine diet, which includes limiting or avoiding high-histamine foods and incorporating whole, nutritious foods, including:

- Fruits except for citrus, strawberries, and avocados

- Vegetables except for spinach, tomatoes, and eggplant

- Herbs

- Grains, such as rice, pasta, oats, quinoa

- Unprocessed meat

- Nut-based milk

- Healthy oils, like olive and canola

- Egg yolks

In addition, there is evidence that how you cook your food can affect the histamine levels in foods. For example, frying and grilling tend to increase histamine levels, while boiling tends to maintain or decrease levels.

Processed Foods and Their Impact on Skin Health

Processed foods can have a negative effect on your skin. Here are some ways in which processed foods can affect your skin:

Excess sugar in the diet, which often comes from highly refined grains and sugars in processed foods, can encourage the degradation of collagen and elastin in your skin, leading to a loss of firmness, loss of elasticity, and an onslaught of premature sagging and wrinkles.

Processed foods are often higher in unhealthy saturated fats and even trans fats, which can stimulate oil production in your skin, leading to clogged pores and increased acne breakouts.

Processed foods are high in added sugars, which are linked to excess "glycation" in the skin, leading to sagging skin.

Processed meats contain high amounts of saturated fats and nitrates that lead to inflammation.

Fatty meats, cow's milk and other dairy products, whey protein, microwave meals, mayonnaise, baked goods, and pretzels are some of the worst foods for your skin.

Alcohol and Caffeine: Their Effects on Vitiligo

Alcohol and caffeine can both influence the condition of vitiligo, where patches of skin lose pigment. Here's how each can potentially affect it:

1. Alcohol:

- Dehydration: Alcohol is a diuretic, which means it increases urine production and can lead to dehydration. Dehydrated skin may worsen existing skin conditions like vitiligo.

- Immune System: Excessive alcohol consumption can weaken the immune system, which plays a role in autoimmune conditions such as vitiligo.

- Vitamin Absorption: Alcohol can interfere with the absorption of essential vitamins needed for healthy skin, potentially impacting conditions like vitiligo.

2. Caffeine:

- Stress and Anxiety: Caffeine can increase cortisol levels (stress hormone), which might aggravate autoimmune conditions like vitiligo.

- Sleep Disturbance: Poor sleep due to caffeine can affect overall skin health and potentially worsen skin conditions.

- Blood Flow: Caffeine can affect blood flow to the skin, which could impact melanocyte function (cells responsible for skin pigmentation).

Recommendations:

- Moderation: It's important to consume alcohol and caffeine in moderation to minimize potential negative effects on skin health, including vitiligo.

- Hydration: Maintaining adequate hydration is crucial, especially when consuming alcohol or caffeine, to counteract dehydration effects.

- Consultation: If you have vitiligo or any skin condition, consulting with a dermatologist can provide personalized advice on managing lifestyle factors like alcohol and caffeine intake.

PART IV
DELICIOUSLY SIMPLE RECIPES
YOU MUST TRY!

BREAKFAST RECIPES FOR VITILIGO

Gluten-free banana pancakes

Ingredients

- 1 large banana

- 2 medium eggs, beaten

- pinch of baking powder (gluten-free if coeliac)

- splash of vanilla extract

- 1 tsp oil

- 25g pecans, roughly chopped

- 125g raspberries

How to Make

- **STEP 1**

In a bowl, mash 1 large banana with a fork until it resembles a thick purée.

- **STEP 2**

Stir in 2 beaten eggs, a pinch of baking powder (gluten-free if coeliac) and a splash of vanilla extract.

- **STEP 3**

Heat a large non-stick frying pan or pancake pan over a medium heat and brush with ½ tsp oil.

- **STEP 4**

Using half the batter, spoon two pancakes into the pan, cook for 1-2 mins each side, then tip onto a plate. Repeat the process with another ½ tsp oil and the remaining batter.

- STEP 5

Top the pancakes with 25g roughly chopped pecans and 125g raspberries.

Green goddess smoothie bowl

Ingredients

- 2 bananas, sliced

- 1 ripe avocado, stoned, peeled and chopped into chunks

- 1 small ripe mango, stoned, peeled and chopped into chunks

- 100g spinach (fresh or frozen)

- 250ml milk (unsweetened almond or coconut milk works well)

- 1 tbsp unsweetened almond or peanut butter

- 1 tbsp clear honey, agave or maple syrup (optional)

For the seed mix

- 1 tbsp chia seeds

- 1 tbsp linseeds

- 4 tbsp pumpkin seeds

- 4 tbsp sunflower seeds

- 4 tbsp coconut flakes

- 4 tbsp flaked almonds

- ¼ tsp ground cinnamon

- 2 tbsp clear honey, agave or maple syrup

To serve

- 175g mixed fresh fruit, chopped (we used banana, mango, raspberries and blueberries)

How to Make

- STEP 1

Slice the bananas and arrange over a small baking tray lined with parchment. Freeze for 2 hrs until solid. (You can now transfer the banana slices to a freezer bag and freeze for 3 months, or continue with the recipe.)

- STEP 2

For the seed mix, heat oven to 180C/160C fan/gas 4 and line a baking tray with parchment. Tip the seeds, coconut and almonds into a bowl, add the cinnamon and drizzle over the honey, agave or maple syrup. Toss until everything is well coated, then scatter over the baking tray in an even layer.

Bake for 10-15 mins, stirring every 5 mins or so, until the seeds are lightly toasted. Leave to cool. Will keep in an airtight container for up to 1 month.

- STEP 3

Put the avocado, mango, spinach, milk, nut butter, frozen banana slices and honey (if using) in a blender and whizz to a thick smoothie consistency – you may have to scrape down the sides with a spoon a few times. Divide between two bowls and arrange the fruit on top. Scatter 1-2 tbsp of the seed mix over each bowl and eat straight away.

Summer porridge

Ingredients

- 300ml almond milk

- 200g blueberries

- ½ tbsp maple syrup

- 2 tbsp chia seeds

- 100g jumbo oats

- 1 kiwi fruit, cut into slices

- 50g pomegranate seeds

- 2 tsp mixed seeds

How to Make

- STEP 1

In a blender, blitz the milk, blueberries and maple syrup until the milk turns purple. Put the chia and oats in a mixing bowl, pour in the blueberry milk and stir very well. Leave to soak for 5 mins, stirring occasionally, until the liquid has absorbed, and the oats and chia thicken and swell.

- STEP 2

Stir again, then divide between two bowls. Arrange the fruit on top, then sprinkle over the mixed seeds. Will keep in the fridge for 1 day. Add the toppings just before serving.

Vegan breakfast muffins

Ingredients

- 150g muesli mix

- 50g light brown soft sugar

- 160g plain flour

- 1 tsp baking powder

- 250ml sweetened soy milk

- 1 apple, peeled and grated

- 2 tbsp grapeseed oil

- 3 tbsp nut butter (we used almond)

- 4 tbsp demerara sugar

- 50g pecans, roughly chilled

How to Make

- STEP 1

Heat the oven to 200C/180C fan/gas 6. Line a muffin tin with cases. Mix 100g muesli with the light brown sugar, flour and baking powder in a bowl. Combine the milk, apple, oil and 2 tbsp nut butter in a jug, then stir into the dry mixture. Divide equally between the cases. Mix the remaining muesli with the demerara sugar, remaining nut butter and the pecans, and spoon over the muffins.

• STEP 2

Bake for 25-30 mins or until the muffins are risen and golden. Will keep for two to three days in an airtight container or freeze for one month. Refresh in the oven before serving.

Crumpets

Ingredients

- 2½ tsp dried yeast

- 240ml warm milk

- 2 tbsp unsalted butter, melted

- 2tsp sea salt

- 2tsp caster sugar

- 470g plain flour

- ½ tsp baking powder dissolved in 60ml warm water

- vegetable oil, to grease

- butter or cheese, to serve

How to Make

- STEP 1

Stir together the yeast and 240ml warm water in a bowl and leave to stand for 5-10 mins. Add the warm milk, butter, salt and sugar, then tip in the flour and stir until smooth. Leave to stand for 30 mins.

- STEP 2

Dissolve the baking powder in a little water, then leave to rise for 20-30 mins.

• STEP 3

Oil a heavy-based frying pan with a little vegetable oil and heat over medium-low heat. Lightly oil four 9cm crumpet rings. Spoon batter into the rings so it comes halfway up the sides. Reduce heat to low, cover with a lid, or an upturned deep frying pan to give the crumpets space to rise. Cook until the tops look dry, about 10-12 mins.

• STEP 4

Flip them over and cook for 5 mins until golden and firm. Repeat with the remaining batter. Serve toasted with butter or topped with cheese, melted under the grill.

Raspberry coconut porridge

Ingredients

- 100g rolled porridge oats (not instant)
- 25g creamed coconut, chopped
- 200g frozen raspberries
- 125g pot coconut yogurt (we used COYO)
- a few mint leaves, to serve (optional)

How to Make

- STEP 1

Tip the oats and creamed coconut into a large bowl, pour on 800ml cold water, cover and leave to soak overnight.

- STEP 2

The next day, tip the contents of the bowl into a saucepan and cook over a medium heat, stirring frequently, for 5 -10 mins until the oats are cooked. Add the raspberries to the pan with the yogurt and allow to thaw and melt into the oats off the heat. Reserve half for the next day and spoon the remainder into bowls. Top each portion with mint leaves, if you like.

Chocolate crumpets

Ingredients

- 300ml milk

- 200g plain flour

- 2 tbsp cocoa powder

- 1 tsp fast-action dried yeast

- 2 tbsp golden caster sugar

- 2 tbsp vegetable oil, plus extra for the pan

How to Make

- STEP 1

Heat 300ml of the milk in a pan until it just starts to bubble around the edges, then leave it to cool until it is tepid.

- STEP 2

Measure out the flour and then put 3 tbsp back into the bag. Add the cocoa, yeast and sugar, and then stir in the milk, a little at a time, until you have a smooth batter. Cover and leave to rise in a warm place for 1hr-1hr 30 mins or until doubled in size and very bubbly. Stir in a little more milk if the batter is very thick – if it is too thick the bubbles won't rise to the surface as well.

- **STEP 3**

When risen, add the remaining 50ml milk to the batter to let it down a little, then heat the grill to high. Lightly oil the insides of 4 x 9cm metal crumpet rings or metal cook's rings. Heat a large non-stick frying pan or griddle pan over a low-medium heat, add 1 tbsp oil and put the rings in the pan. Spoon the batter into the rings until they are half full. Let the crumpets cook slowly for about 10 mins or until the mixture has set and the bubbles on top have all popped. Lift the rings away carefully. Repeat with the remaining mixture.

- **STEP 4**

If you now want to grill the crumpets, transfer the pan (if it has a heatproof handle) to the grill and cook until the tops are golden brown. If the pan doesn't have a heatproof handle, transfer the crumpets to a baking sheet and grill them on that instead. Can be made up to a day ahead or frozen until ready to grill and serve.

Beetroot pancakes

Ingredients

- 3 small cooked whole beetroot, chopped

- 50ml milk

- 200g self raising flour

- 1 tsp baking powder

- 2 tbsp maple syrup

- ½ tsp vanilla extract

- 3 eggs

- 25g butter, melted plus extra for frying

To serve (optional)

- 200g frozen mixed berries

- 2 tbsp blackcurrant jam

- 100g Greek yogurt

How to Make

- STEP 1

Put the beetroot in a jug with the milk and blend with a stick blender until smooth. Pour into a bowl with the rest of the pancake Ingredients and whisk until smooth and vibrant purple.

- STEP 2

Put a small knob of butter in a large non-stick frying pan and heat over a medium-low heat until melted and foamy. Now create 3 or 4 pancakes each made from 2 tbsp of the batter. Cook for 2-3 mins then flip over and cook for a further minute until cooked through. Repeat with any remaining batter. Heat oven to lowest setting and keep the pancakes warm in there until needed.

- STEP 3

Serve with your favourite pancake toppings or make a simple compote by simmering frozen berries in with 1 tbsp blackcurrant jam until bubbling and syrupy (about 5-10 mins). In a small bowl stir together the remaining jam and the yogurt. Stack the cooked pancakes with the yogurt and pour the warm berry compote over the top.

Berry omelette

Ingredients

- 1 large egg

- 1 tbsp skimmed milk

- 3 pinches of cinnamon

- ½ tsp rapeseed oil

- 100g cottage cheese

- 175g chopped strawberry, blueberries and raspberries

Instructions

- STEP 1

Beat egg with milk and cinnamon. Heat oil in a 20cm non-stick frying pan and pour in the egg mixture, swirling to evenly cover the base. Cook for a few mins until set and golden underneath. There's no need to flip it over.

- STEP 2

Place on a plate, spread over cheese, then scatter with berries. Roll up and serve.

Creamy smoked haddock & saffron kedgeree

Ingredients

- 300g basmati rice

- 50g butter

- 3 hard-boiled eggs, shelled and halved

- 200ml double cream

- 500g naturally smoked haddock, skin removed

- 100ml white wine

- 1tsp cayenne pepper

- pinch saffron strands

- 1 tbsp mild curry powder

- freshly grated nutmeg

- small handful flat-leaf parsley, chopped

- 1 lemon, cut into wedges, to serve

Instructions

- STEP 1

Cook basmati rice, leave to cool. Heat oven to 160C/140C fan/gas 3. Grease a large ovenproof dish with some of the butter. Push the egg yolks through a sieve and roughly chop the whites.

- STEP 2

Gently heat the cream in a frying pan until just below boiling point, then add the fish. Cover and poach for 4 mins. Place the wine in a pan with the saffron and warm to infuse. In a large bowl, mix together the rice, cayenne, curry powder, nutmeg, seasoning, chopped egg whites and saffron-infused wine. Lift the fish out of the cream and flake into the bowl – removing any bones as you find them. Scrape in the cream and gently mix together once more.

- STEP 3

Tip everything into the buttered dish and dot the top with the remaining butter. Bake to heat through for 20 mins, then serve scattered with the parsley and sieved egg yolk, with lemon wedges on the side.

Kale & salmon kedgeree

Ingredients

- 300g brown rice

- 2 salmon fillets (about 280g)

- 4 eggs

- 1 tbsp vegetable oil

- 1 onion, finely chopped

- 100g curly kale, stalks removed, roughly chopped

- 1 garlic clove, crushed

- 1 tbsp curry powder

- 1 tsp turmeric

- zest and juice 1 lemon

Instructions

- STEP 1

Cook the rice following pack instructions. Meanwhile, season the salmon and steam over a pan of simmering water for 8 mins or until just cooked. Keep the pan of water on the heat, add the eggs and boil for 6 mins, then run under cold water.

- STEP 2

Heat the oil in a large frying pan or wok, add the onion and cook for 5 mins. Throw in the kale and cook, stirring, for 5 mins. Add the garlic, curry powder, turmeric and rice, season and stir until heated through.

- STEP 3

Peel and quarter the eggs. Flake the salmon and gently fold through the rice, then divide between plates and top with the eggs. Sprinkle over the lemon zest and squeeze over a little juice before serving.

Cured salmon

Ingredients

- 1 tbsp cracked black pepper

- 75g muscovado sugar

- 60g sea salt flakes

- 1 filleted side of very fresh salmon (about 800g), skin on

For the dill & lemon cream cheese

- 200g full-fat cream cheese, at room temperature

- small bunch of dill, finely chopped

- ½ unwaxed lemon, zested and juiced, plus extra wedges to serve

For the pickle

- 1 small cucumber

- 1 small red onion, finely sliced

- pinch of caster sugar

- 3 tbsp white wine vinegar

To serve

- selection of toasted bagels

- sliced rye bread

- small pot of salmon caviar

- caper berries or capers, drained

Instructions

- STEP 1

Up to four days but at least two days before serving the salmon, mix the pepper, sugar and salt together. Pat the salmon dry with kitchen paper and run your hands over the flesh to find any stray bones – use tweezers to pull these out, if needed. Lay the salmon in a dish, skin-side down, and pack the salt mix over the flesh. Cover the fish with a board or tray weighed down with a few heavy cans or jars. Transfer to the fridge for at least two days or up to four, turning the fillet about every 12 hrs.

- STEP 2

To make the dill cream cheese, beat all of the Ingredients together and set aside. This can be made up to a day ahead and chilled.

- STEP 3

To make the pickle, cut the cucumber in half lengthways, scoop out the seeds using a spoon, and slice into thin half-moons. Toss the cucumber with the red onion and a generous pinch of salt in a colander, then set aside for 30 mins to soften. Transfer the vegetables to a bowl or jar and top up with the sugar and vinegar. Can be eaten immediately or made up to two days ahead and chilled.

• STEP 4

Lift the salmon out of the curing mixture and wipe off any excess seasoning using kitchen paper. Put the fish on a large serving board and carve into thin slices. Serve with the bagels and rye bread, dill & lemon cream cheese, the pickle, salmon caviar, capers and lemon wedges.

Strawberry-Pineapple Smoothie

Ingredients

1 cup frozen strawberries

1 cup chopped fresh pineapple

¾ cup chilled unsweetened almond milk, plus more if needed

1 tablespoon almond butter

How to Make

Combine strawberries, pineapple, almond milk and almond butter in a blender. Process until smooth, adding more almond milk, if needed, for desired consistency. Serve immediately.

Chickpea & Potato Hash

Ingredients

4 cups frozen shredded hash brown potatoes

2 cups finely chopped baby spinach

½ cup finely chopped onion

1 tablespoon minced fresh ginger

1 tablespoon curry powder

½ teaspoon salt

¼ cup extra-virgin olive oil

1 15-ounce can chickpeas, rinsed

1 cup chopped zucchini

4 large eggs

How to Make

1. Combine potatoes, spinach, onion, ginger, curry powder and salt in a large bowl.
2. Heat oil in a large nonstick skillet over medium-high heat. Add the potato mixture and press into a layer. Cook, without stirring, until crispy and golden brown on the bottom, 3 to 5 minutes.
3. Reduce heat to medium-low. Fold in chickpeas and zucchini, breaking up chunks of potato, until just combined. Press back into an even layer. Carve out 4 "wells" in the mixture. Break eggs, one at a time, into a cup and slip one into each indentation. Cover and continue cooking until the eggs are set, 4 to 5 minutes for soft-set yolks.

Cheddar and Zucchini Frittata

Ingredients

1 cup refrigerated or frozen egg product, thawed or 4 eggs

½ cup finely shredded reduced-fat cheddar cheese

2 tablespoons snipped fresh flat-leaf parsley

¼ teaspoon ground black pepper

⅛ teaspoon salt

2 teaspoons olive oil

12 ounces zucchini, halved lengthwise and sliced

4 green onions, sliced

How to Make

1. Position a rack in the upper third of the oven and preheat to 450 degrees F. In a medium bowl, whisk together eggs, cheese, half of the parsley, the pepper and salt. Set aside.
2. In a 9- to 10-inch ovenproof skillet, heat olive oil over medium-high heat. Add zucchini and green onions; cook 5 to 8 minutes or just until tender, stirring frequently.
3. Carefully pour the egg mixture over the vegetables. Reduce heat to medium. As mixture sets, run a spatula around the edge of the skillet, lifting egg mixture so uncooked portion flows underneath. Continue cooking and lifting edges about 5 minutes or until egg mixture is almost set (surface will be moist). Reduce heat as necessary to prevent overbrowning.
4. Place the skillet in the oven. Bake about 5 minutes or until the frittata is firm and the top is golden. Sprinkle with remaining 2

tablespoons parsley. Cut into wedges. Serve warm.

Spinach & Feta Scrambled Egg Pitas

Ingredients

1 tablespoon extra-virgin olive oil

1 (10 ounce) block frozen chopped spinach, thawed, drained and squeezed dry

Pinch salt

8 large eggs, beaten

¼ cup finely crumbled feta cheese

Freshly ground pepper to taste

8 teaspoons sun-dried tomato tapenade or sun-dried tomato pesto

4 whole-wheat pitas (5-inch), cut in half, warmed if desired (see Tip)

How to Make

1. Heat oil in a large nonstick skillet over medium heat. Add spinach and salt and cook until steaming hot, stirring occasionally. Add eggs and cook, stirring the eggs as they set, until they form soft curds and are just moist, 4 to 5 minutes. Add feta and pepper and cook until set.
2. Spread tapenade (or pesto) inside pita pockets, 2 teaspoons per pita. Divide the egg mixture among the pitas.

Baked Eggs in Tomato Sauce with Kale

Ingredients

1 tablespoon extra-virgin olive oil

3 10-ounce packages frozen chopped kale, thawed, drained and squeezed dry (9 cups)

½ teaspoon salt, divided

¼ teaspoon ground pepper, divided

1 25-ounce jar low-sodium marinara sauce or 3 cups canned low-sodium tomato sauce

8 large eggs

How to Make

1. Preheat oven to 350 degrees F.
2. Heat oil in a 10-inch cast-iron skillet or nonstick ovenproof skillet over medium heat. Add kale, season with 1/4 teaspoon salt and 1/8 teaspoon pepper, and sauté for 2 minutes. Stir in

marinara (or tomato) sauce and bring to a simmer.

3. Make 8 wells in the sauce with the back of a spoon and carefully crack an egg into each well. Season the eggs with the remaining 1/4 teaspoon salt and 1/8 teaspoon pepper.

4. Transfer the pan to the oven and bake until the egg whites are set and the yolks are still soft, about 20 minutes.

LUNCH RECIPES FOR VITILIGO

Vegetarian lasagne

Ingredients

- 3 red peppers, cut into large chunks

- 2 aubergines, cut into ½ cm thick slices

- 8 tbsp olive oil, plus extra for the dish

- 300g lasagne sheets

- 125g mozzarella

- handful cherry tomatoes, halved

For the tomato sauce

- 1 tbsp olive oil

- 2 onions, finely chopped

- 2 garlic cloves, sliced

- 1 carrot, roughly chopped

- 2 tbsp tomato purée

- 200ml white wine

- 3 x 400g cans chopped tomatoes

- 1 bunch of basil, leaves picked

For the white sauce

- 85g butter

- 85g plain flour

- 750ml milk

How to Make

- STEP 1

To make the tomato sauce, heat the olive oil in a saucepan. Add the onions, garlic and carrot. Cook for 5-7 mins over a medium heat until softened. Turn up the heat a little and stir in the tomato purée. Cook for 1 min, pour in the white wine, then cook for 5 mins until this has reduced by two-thirds. Pour over the chopped tomatoes and add the basil leaves. Bring to the boil then simmer for 20 mins. Leave to cool then whizz in a food processor. Will keep, cooled, in the fridge for up to three days or frozen for three months.

- STEP 2

To make the white sauce, melt the butter in a saucepan, stir in the plain flour, then cook for 2 mins. Slowly whisk in the milk, then bring to the boil, stirring. Turn down the heat, then cook until the sauce starts to thicken and coats the back of a wooden spoon. Will keep, cooled, in the fridge for up to three days or frozen for three months.

- STEP 3

Heat the oven to 200C/180C fan/gas 6. Lightly oil two large baking trays and add the peppers and aubergines. Toss with the olive oil, season well, then roast for 25 mins until lightly browned.

- STEP 4

Reduce the oven to 180C/160C fan/gas 4. Lightly oil a 30 x 20cm ovenproof dish. Arrange a layer of the vegetables on the bottom, then pour over a third of the tomato sauce. Top with a layer of lasagne sheets, then drizzle over a quarter of the white sauce. Repeat until you have three layers of pasta.

- STEP 5

Spoon the remaining white sauce over the pasta, making sure the whole surface is covered, then scatter over the mozzarella and cherry tomatoes. Bake for 45 mins until bubbling and golden.

Tomato, watermelon & feta salad with mint dressing

Ingredients

- 2 tbsp olive oil

- 1 tbsp red wine vinegar

- ¼ tsp chilli flakes

- 2 tbsp chopped mint

- 4 tomatoes, chopped

- 500g/1lb 2oz watermelon, cut into chunks

- 200g pack feta cheese, crumbled

How to Make

- STEP 1

Make the dressing by mixing the oil, vinegar, chilli flakes and mint with some seasoning.

- STEP 2

Put the tomatoes and watermelon in a bowl. Pour over the dressing and leave to stand for 10 mins to allow the fruit to get really juicy. Gently stir through the feta, then serve.

Asparagus & lentil salad with cranberries & crumbled feta

Ingredients

- 1 garlic clove

- 125g puy lentils

- 100g pack fine asparagus tips

- 3 spring onions, finely sliced

- 25g dried cranberries

- 1 tbsp extra virgin rapeseed oil, plus a little extra (optional)

- 2 tsp organic apple cider vinegar

- 140g cherry tomatoes, halved

- 50g feta (read back of pack for vegetarian option)

How to Make

- STEP 1

Finely grate the garlic and put in a bowl. Boil the lentils for 25 mins, and put the asparagus in a steamer over them for the last 5 mins until just tender.

• STEP 2

Meanwhile, put the onions, cranberries, oil and vinegar in the bowl with the garlic and stir well. When the lentils are ready, drain and toss them into the dressing with the tomatoes. Tip into plastic containers (for a packed lunch), or onto plates, then top with the asparagus and crumble over the feta. Drizzle with a little extra oil, if you like.

Roasted summer vegetable casserole

Ingredients

- 3 tbsp olive oil

- 1 garlic bulb, halved through the middle

- 2 large courgettes, thickly sliced

- 1 large red onion, sliced

- 1 aubergine, halved and sliced on the diagonal

- 2 large tomatoes, quartered

- 200g new potatoes, scrubbed and halved

- 1 red pepper, deseeded and cut into chunky pieces

- 400g can chopped tomatoes

- 0.5 small pack parsley, chopped

How to Make

- STEP 1

Heat oven to 200C/180C fan/gas 6 and put the oil in a roasting tin. Tip in the garlic and all the fresh veg, then toss with your hands to coat in the oil. Season well and roast for 45 mins.

- STEP 2

Remove the garlic from the roasting tin and squeeze out the softened cloves all over the veg, stirring to evenly distribute. In a medium pan, simmer the chopped tomatoes until bubbling, season well and stir through the roasted veg in the tin. Scatter over the parsley and serve.

Sweet potato jackets with pomegranate & celeriac slaw

Ingredients

- 2 sweet potatoes (about 195g each)

- 90g pomegranate seeds

- 8 walnut halves, broken

- small handful coriander, chopped

- 120g pot bio yogurt

For the slaw

- 1 small red onion, halved and thinly sliced

- 160g peeled celeriac, thinly sliced into matchsticks

- 2 celery sticks, chopped

- 1 tbsp lemon juice

- 1 tbsp rapeseed oil

- 2 tsp balsamic vinegar

- 0.5 - 1 tsp English mustard powder (optional)

- 2 tbsp chopped parsley

How to Make

- STEP 1

Heat oven to 200C/180C fan/gas 6. Roast the sweet potatoes for 35-40 mins until a knife slides in easily.

- STEP 2

Meanwhile, pour boiling water over the onion and leave for 5 mins, then rinse under the cold tap and pat dry with kitchen paper. Tip into a bowl and add the celeriac and celery with all but 4 tbsp yogurt along with the remaining slaw Ingredients and toss together.

- STEP 3

Cut into the potatoes and gently squeeze to open them. Top with the remaining yogurt, pomegranate and walnuts. Scatter over the coriander. Serve with the slaw.

Bean, tomato & watercress salad

Ingredients

- 2 x 400g can cannellini beans

- 100g watercress

- 1 lemon, zested and juiced

- 250g pack sundried tomatoes and olives

How to Make

- STEP 1

Drain and rinse the beans, then combine in a bowl with the watercress, zest and juice of the lemon, tomatoes and olives, including the oil from the pack. Toss well and season to taste.

Lemon roast vegetables with yogurt tahini & pomegranate

Ingredients

- 1 red pepper, deseeded and chopped

- 1 aubergine, diced

- 1 red onion, halved and thinly sliced

- 1 unwaxed lemon, 1/4 finely chopped (skin and all), the rest juiced

- 1 tbsp rapeseed oil, plus extra to drizzle (optional)

- 400g can chickpeas in water, drained

- 1 garlic clove

- 2 tbsp tahini

- 3 tbsp natural bio yogurt

- seeds from ½ a pomegranate

- ⅓ small pack parsley or coriander, chopped

How to Make

- STEP 1

Heat oven to 240C/220C fan/gas 7. Put the vegetables and chopped lemon in a large flameproof roasting tin and drizzle with 1 tbsp oil. Massage into the veg so they are all well coated, then put the tin on the hob and fry, stirring, for 5 mins until starting to char. Stir in two handfuls of the chickpeas, and roast in the oven for 15 mins.

- STEP 2

Put the rest of the chickpeas in a bowl with the garlic, tahini, yogurt, lemon juice and 3 tbsp water, and blitz with a stick blender until really smooth and thick.

- STEP 3

Spoon the yogurt tahini onto two plates and top with the roasted veg, pomegranate seeds and parsley. Season with black pepper and a drizzle of extra oil, if you like.

BBQ mackerel

Ingredients

- 3 tbsp extra-virgin olive oil

- 4 small whole mackerel, gutted and cleaned

For the drizzle

- 1 large red chilli, deseeded and finely chopped

- 1 small garlic clove, finely chopped

- small knob fresh root ginger, finely chopped

- 2 tsp honey

- 2 limes, zested and juiced

- 1 tsp sesame oil

- 1 tsp Thai fish sauce

How to Make

- STEP 1

Light the barbecue and allow the flames to die down until the ashes have gone white with heat. Make the drizzle by whisking 2 tbsp olive oil and all the other Ingredients together in a small bowl, adjusting the ratio of honey and lime to make a sharp sweetness. Season to taste.

- STEP 2

Score each side of the mackerel about 6 times, not quite through to the bone. Brush the fish with the remaining oil and season lightly. Barbecue the mackerel for 5-6 mins on each side until the fish is charred and the eyes have turned white. Spoon the drizzle over the fish and allow to stand for 2-3 mins before serving.

Korean fishcakes with fried eggs & spicy salsa

Ingredients

For the fishcakes

- 4 x loch trout or rainbow trout fillets, skinned and cut into 1cm/ 1/2in pieces (about 450g/1lb fish)

- 2 tsp finely grated ginger

- 1 fat garlic clove, crushed

- 1 tsp light soy sauce

- bunch spring onions, thinly sliced

- 1 large egg white, beaten until frothy

- 2 tbsp rice flour

- 2 ½ tbsp vegetable oil, for frying

For the salad

- 1 pointed or small white cabbage, cored and finely shredded (about 350g/12oz)

- 100g radishes, thinly sliced

- 2 tbsp Chinese rice vinegar

- 1 tbsp sesame oil, plus 2 tsp to serve

- 1 tsp gochujang, plus 2 top to serve (see tip)

- 1 tsp golden caster sugar

- 1 garlic clove, crushed

- 2 tsp light soy sauce

- 4 medium eggs

- 1 tbsp sesame seeds, toasted

- 1 red chilli, finely sliced, to serve (optional)

How to Make

- STEP 1

For the fishcakes, mix the fish with the ginger, garlic, soy and half the spring onions. Stir in the egg white and rice flour.

- STEP 2

Toss the cabbage and radishes with the vinegar, 1 tbsp sesame oil, 1 tsp gochujang, the sugar and garlic. Set aside. Stir together the remaining sesame oil, gochujang and the soy sauce to make a drizzling sauce for later.

- STEP 3

Heat 1 tbsp oil in a large, non-stick frying pan. Split the fish mixture into eight, then spoon four into the pan, pressing the mix to make cakes about 8cm across. Fry for 2 mins each side until just cooked through and golden. Add another 1 tbsp oil to the pan and repeat with the remaining fish. Keep warm in a low oven.

- STEP 4

Add the remaining oil to the pan. Fry the eggs for 2-3 mins until crisp but with a runny yolk. Serve the fishcakes with the cabbage, and top with the egg and sesame seeds. Scatter with the rest of the spring onions, red chilli (if using) and some of the chilli sesame drizzle.

Classic lasagne

Ingredients

- 2 olive oil, plus extra for the dish

- 750g lean beef mince

- 90g pack prosciutto

- 800g passata or half our basic tomato sauce

- 200ml hot beef stock

- nutmeg

- 300g fresh lasagne sheets

- white sauce (find a recipe in the direction, or use shop-bought)

- 125g ball mozzarella, torn into thin strips

How to Make

- STEP 1

To make the meat sauce, heat 2 tbsp olive oil in a frying pan and cook 750g lean beef mince in two batches for about 10 mins until browned all over.

- STEP 2

Finely chop 4 slices of prosciutto from a 90g pack, then stir through the meat mixture.

- STEP 3

Pour over 800g passata or half our basic tomato sauce recipe and 200ml hot beef stock. Add a little grated nutmeg, then season.

- STEP 4

Bring up to the boil, then simmer for 30 mins until the sauce looks rich.

- STEP 5

Heat the oven to 180C/160C fan/gas 4 and lightly oil an ovenproof dish (about 30 x 20cm).

- STEP 6

Spoon one third of the meat sauce into the dish, then cover with some fresh lasagne sheets from a 300g pack. Drizzle over roughly 130g ready-made or homemade white sauce.

- STEP 7

Repeat until you have three layers of pasta. Cover with the remaining 390g white sauce, making sure you can't see any pasta poking through.

- STEP 8

Scatter 125g torn mozzarella over the top.

- STEP 9

Arrange the rest of the prosciutto on top. Bake for 45 mins until the top is bubbling and lightly browned.

Haddock in tomato basil sauce

Ingredients

- 1 tbsp olive oil

- 1 onion, thinly sliced

- 1 small aubergine, about 250g/9oz, roughly chopped

- ½ tsp ground paprika

- 2 garlic cloves, crushed

- 400g can chopped tomato

- 1 tsp dark or light muscovado sugar

- 8 large basil leaves, plus a few extra for sprinkling

- 4 4x175g/6oz firm skinless white fish fillets, such as haddock

How to Make

- STEP 1

Heat the olive oil in a large non-stick frying pan and stirfry the onion and aubergine. After about 4 minutes the vegetables will start to turn golden but won't be soft yet, so cover with a lid and let the vegetables steam-fry in their own juices for 6 minutes – this helps them to soften without needing to add any extra oil.

- STEP 2

Stir in the paprika, garlic, tomatoes and sugar with 1/2 tsp salt and cook for another 8-10 minutes, stirring, until onion and aubergine are tender.

- STEP 3

Scatter in the basil leaves then nestle the fish in the sauce, cover the pan and cook for 6-8 minutes until the fish flakes when tested with a knife and the flesh is firm but still moist. Tear over the rest of the basil and serve with a salad and crusty bread.

Antipasti salmon

Ingredients

- 100g sundried tomatoes in oil, drained and finely chopped

- small handful of basil, finely chopped, plus a few whole basil leaves

- small handful of dill, finely chopped, plus a few dill fronds to serve

- 2 tbsp capers, drained and rinsed

- 2 garlic cloves, crushed

- 1 lemon, zested and sliced

- 150g butter, softened

- 600g side of salmon, descaled and pin bones removed

- 3 tbsp pitted black olives

- 100g griddled artichoke hearts, drained and roughly chopped

How to Make

- STEP 1

Put the tomatoes, half the herbs, 1 tbsp capers, the garlic, lemon zest and butter in a bowl and mash together with a spoon. Alternatively, tip into a food processor and blitz until combined. The flavoured butter will keep, chilled, for up to two days.

- STEP 2

Layer a sheet of baking parchment large enough to loosely wrap the salmon over an equally-sized sheet of foil. Place the salmon on top, then cut the fish into portions, without cutting all the way through to the skin, so the fillet remains intact. Make the portions as big or small as you like, depending on how many you're feeding. Spread the flavoured butter over the salmon, then top with the remaining capers, the lemon slices, olives and artichokes. Wrap the foil and parchment over the salmon and scrunch the ends to seal, creating a loose parcel.

• STEP 3

To bake the salmon, heat the oven to 200C/180C fan/gas 6. Put the parcel on a baking tray and cook for 30 mins, then leave to stand for a few minutes before unwrapping. Alternatively, light the barbecue, wait for the flames to die down, put the parcel directly on the grill and cook for 8-15 mins, or until the salmon is cooked through. Check the salmon is cooked by pushing the flesh with a fork – it should easily flake. Serve on a platter, scattered with the remaining herbs and the buttery juices poured over.

Sticky onion & cheddar quiche

Ingredients

- 25g butter

- 500g small onion, (about 5 in total), halved and finely sliced

- 2 eggs

- 284ml pot double cream

- 140g mature cheddar, coarsely grated

For the pastry

- 280g plain flour, plus extra for dusting

- 140g cold butter

How to Make

- STEP 1

To make the pastry, tip the flour and butter into a bowl, then rub together with your fingertips until completely mixed and crumbly. Add 8 tbsp cold water, then bring everything together with your hands until just combined. Roll into a ball and use straight away or chill for up to 2 days. The pastry can also be frozen for up to a month.

- STEP 2

Roll out the pastry on a lightly floured surface to a round about 5cm larger than a 25cm tin. Use your rolling pin to lift it up, then drape over the tart case so there is an overhang of pastry on the sides. Using a small ball of pastry scraps, push the pastry into the corners of the tin (see picture, above left). Chill in the fridge or freezer for 20 mins.

• STEP 3

Heat oven to 200C/fan 180C/gas 6. While the pastry is chilling, heat the butter in a pan and cook the onions for 20 mins, stirring occasionally, until they become sticky and golden. Remove from the heat.

• STEP 4

Lightly prick the base of the tart with a fork, line the tart case with a large circle of greaseproof paper or foil, then fill with baking beans. Blind-bake the tart for 20 mins, remove the paper and beans, then continue to cook for 5-10 mins until biscuit brown.

• STEP 5

Meanwhile, beat the eggs in a bowl, then gradually add the cream. Stir in the onions and half the cheese, then season with salt and pepper. Carefully tip the filling into the case, sprinkle with the rest of the cheese, then bake for 20-25 mins until set and golden. Leave to cool in the case, trim the edges of the pastry, then remove and serve in slices.

Steamed bass with pak choi

Ingredients

- small piece of ginger, peeled and sliced

- 2 garlic cloves, finely sliced

- 3 spring onions, finely sliced

- 2 tbsp soy sauce

- 1 tbsp sesame oil

- splash of sherry (optional)

- 2 x fillets sea bass

- 2 heads pak choi, quartered

How to Make

- STEP 1

In a small bowl, mix all of the Ingredients, except the fish and the pak choi, together to make a soy mix. Line one tier of a two-tiered bamboo steamer loosely with foil. Lay the fish, skin side up, on the foil and spoon over the soy mix. Place the fish over simmering water and throw the pak choi into the second tier and cover it with a lid. Alternatively, add the pak choi to the fish layer after 2 mins of cooking – the closer the tier is to the steam, the hotter it is.

- STEP 2

Leave everything to steam for 6-8 mins until the pak choi has wilted and the fish is cooked. Divide the greens between two plates, then carefully lift out the fish. Lift the foil up and drizzle the tasty juices back over the fish.

Mackerel with orange & harissa glaze

Ingredients

- 2 x 300g/10oz mackerel, filleted and skin on or 4 x 75g/3oz mackerel fillets, skin on

- 2 tbsp plain flour

- ½ tsp smoked paprika

- 2 tbsp extra-virgin olive oil

- 1small orange, grated zest and juice

- 1-2 tsp harissa paste (to taste, as brands vary)

- 50g pine nut, toasted

- small bunch coriander, very roughly chopped

How to Make

- STEP 1

Roll the mackerel fillets in the flour sifted with smoked paprika and seasoning. Shake off excess flour and set the fish aside in a single layer.

- STEP 2

Put 1 tbsp of the olive oil, the orange zest and juice and the harissa paste into a small bowl, and whisk together. Heat a frying pan with remaining olive oil until very hot. Fry the fish fillets for 5 mins, first on the skin side, then on the flesh side.

- STEP 3

When the fish is nearly cooked – it should look firm – pour over the orange and harissa glaze, bring to the boil and allow the liquid to bubble until sticky. Sprinkle over the pine nuts and coriander.

DINNER RECIPES FOR VITILIGO

Black bean chilli

Ingredients

2 tbsp olive oil

4 garlic cloves, finely chopped

2 large onions, chopped

3 tbsp sweet pimenton (Spanish paprika) or mild chilli powder

3 tbsp ground cumin

3 tbsp cider vinegar

2 tbsp brown sugar

2 x 400g (2 x 14oz) cans chopped tomatoes

2 x 400g (2 x 14oz) cans black beans, rinsed and drained

a few, or one, of the following to serve: crumbled feta cheese (or a dairy-free alternative), chopped spring onions, sliced radishes, avocado chunks, soured cream

Instructions

STEP 1

In a large pot, heat the olive oil and fry the garlic and onions for 5 mins until almost softened. Add the pimenton and cumin, cook for a few mins, then add the vinegar, sugar, tomatoes and some seasoning. Cook for 10 mins.

STEP 2

Pour in the beans and cook for another 10 mins. Serve with rice and the accompaniments of your choice in small bowls.

One-pot chicken & rice

Ingredients

1 tbsp smoked paprika

1 tbsp ground coriander

2 garlic cloves, finely grated

2 tsp rapeseed oil

600g boneless, skinless chicken thighs, halved

700ml hot vegetable bouillon, made with 2 tsp powder

250g easy-cook brown rice

320g leeks, washed and sliced

1 tsp dried oregano or 1 tbsp fresh thyme

2 bay leaves (optional)

320g mixed frozen vegetables (we used sliced carrots, broccoli florets and sweetcorn)

Instructions

STEP 1

Put the spices, garlic and oil in a large bowl and mix well. Add the chicken and turn in the mixture until well coated. Heat a large non-stick pan that has a lid, then fry the chicken, uncovered (without extra oil) over a medium-high heat for 5 mins until browned, turning the chicken halfway to brown on both sides. Remove from the pan and set aside on a plate.

STEP 2

Pour the bouillon into the pan, stirring well to incorporate any garlicky bits that may have stuck to the base of the pan, then stir in the rice, leeks, oregano or thyme and bay, if using. Lay the chicken on top, then cover the pan and bring to the boil. Turn down the heat and simmer for 20 mins.

STEP 3

Stir in the frozen vegetables, then cover and simmer for about 5 mins to heat through. Leave to stand for about 5-10 mins, then lightly mix and serve.

Roast chicken with lemon & rosemary roots

Ingredients

4 large carrots (about 400g), cut into big chunks

1 celeriac (about 575g peeled weight), cut into roastie-sized chunks

1 large swede (550g unpeeled), quartered and cut into thick slices

2 red onions, cut into wedges

1 garlic bulb

2 tbsp rapeseed oil

2 tsp sprigs rosemary leaves and woody stalks separated

1 lemon

1 medium chicken (about 1.4kg)

2 x 200g bags curly kale

Instructions

STEP 1

Heat oven to 200C/180C fan/gas 6. Tip the carrots, celeriac, swede, onions and garlic into a large roasting tin with the oil, rosemary leaves and a grinding of black pepper. Toss well and roast for 5-10 mins while you get the chicken ready.

STEP 2

Grate the zest and squeeze the juice from the lemon, set aside and put the lemon shells and the woody stalks from the rosemary inside the chicken. Stir the veg, scatter over the lemon zest and drizzle over the juice, then sit the chicken on top of the veg and roast for 1-1 1/4 hrs until the chicken is tender but still moist. Take the chicken from the oven and leave to rest for 10 mins. Keep the veg in the oven and steam the bags of kale.

STEP 3

Squeeze the garlic from the skins, carve the chicken and serve with the vegetables.

Lemony chicken stew with giant couscous

Ingredients

1 tbsp olive oil

2 onions, chopped

500g skinless boneless chicken thighs, each cut into 2-3 chunks

3 tbsp tagine paste or 2 tbsp ras el hanout

2 x 400g cans tomato with chopped mixed olives

small handful fresh oregano, leaves picked and chopped

2 preserved lemons, flesh removed, skin rinsed and finely chopped

2 tbsp clear honey

1 chicken stock cube

200g giant couscous

handful parsley, chopped

Instructions

STEP 1

Heat the oil in a large flameproof casserole dish with a lid. Add the onions and cook for 10 mins until starting to caramelise. Push the onions to one side of the dish and add the chicken. Cook over a high heat for 5 mins or so until the chicken is browning.

STEP 2

Add the tagine paste, tomatoes, oregano, preserved lemons and honey, and crumble in the stock cube. Fill one of the tomato cans halfway with water and pour this into the dish. Season with a little salt and plenty of black pepper. Give everything a good stir, then cover with a lid and simmer for 40 mins, on a gentle bubble, or for up to 4 hrs over a very low heat if you're eating at different times.

STEP 3

Add the couscous 10 mins before you're ready to serve, cover and simmer for 10 mins or until cooked. If you're eating at different times, scoop your portion into a pan, add 50g couscous and cook in the same way. Stir in some parsley just before serving.

Vegetarian carbonara

Ingredients

4 medium courgettes (use a mix of yellow and green if you can get them)

300g spaghetti

3 large egg yolks

160g vegetarian parmesan-style cheese

1 tbsp olive oil

small bunch fresh lemon thyme or thyme, leaves picked

200g chestnut mushrooms, roughly chopped

4 garlic cloves, crushed

small bunch flat-leaf parsley, chopped (optional)

½ lemon, zested and juiced

Instructions

STEP 1

Put a large pan of salted water on to boil. Halve the courgettes lengthways and scoop out and discard the core, then slice the courgettes at an angle into small diagonal pieces. Put the spaghetti in the pan of boiling water and cook following pack instructions.

STEP 2

To make the creamy carbonara sauce, put the egg yolks in a bowl, add half of the grated cheese, and mix with a fork. Add up to 3 tbsp water to make the sauce less thick. Season and set aside.

STEP 3

Heat a large frying pan on a medium to high heat and pour in a little olive oil. Fry the courgette slices and thyme leaves with a good grinding of black pepper for a minute or two until the courgette starts to soften, then add the mushrooms. Fry for 2-3 mins until golden and slightly softened. For the last minute of the cooking, add the garlic.

STEP 4

Working quickly, drain the pasta, reserving a little of the cooking water. Toss the pasta in the pan with the courgettes and mushrooms, then remove from the heat and add a ladleful of the reserved cooking water and the egg and cheese sauce. Add the fresh parsley, if using, and the lemon zest and juice, then sprinkle over most of the remaining cheese. Stir everything together quickly to coat the pasta. The egg will cook if the pasta is still hot. If you're worried about it, put back on the heat for 1 min.

STEP 5

Pour in a little more of the cooking water, if needed. You should have a silky and shiny sauce. Season to taste, then sprinkle with a little more cheese to serve. Eat straight away, as the sauce can become thick and stodgy if left for too long.

Healthy fish korma

Ingredients

250g brown basmati rice

2 tsp rapeseed oil

220g brown onions, finely chopped

25g ginger, peeled and finely chopped

1 large courgette, (about 260g), peeled and cut into cubes

2 tsp ground turmeric

1 tbsp ground coriander

1 tsp ground cumin

150ml vegetable stock, made with 1 tsp bouillon powder

2 tbsp ground almonds

100ml coconut or plain bio yogurt

2 x 280g cod loins (4 loins)

For the salad

2 red onions (170g), finely chopped

1 lemon, juiced

30g pack of coriander, finely chopped

1 red chilli, finely chopped

2 small bananas, peeled and sliced

For the salad

2 red onions (170g), finely chopped

1 lemon, juiced

30g pack of coriander, finely chopped

1 red chilli, finely chopped

2 small bananas, peeled and sliced

Instructions

STEP 1

Boil the rice for 25 mins until tender. Meanwhile, heat the oil in a wide, non-stick pan over a medium heat and fry the onions and ginger for 8-10 mins, covered, until softened. Add the courgette, spices and stock, then cover and simmer for 10 mins until the courgette is tender. Remove from the heat.

STEP 2

Blitz the mixture directly in the pan using a hand blender until smooth, then return to a low heat heat and stir in the ground almonds and yogurt.

Smoked salmon soufflés

Ingredients

40g butter

25g plain flour

300ml milk

85g Philadelphia cheese

2 tsp chopped dill

3 large eggs, separated

85g smoked salmon, chopped

zest ½ lemon

To serve

6 tsp crème fraîche

2 large slices smoked salmon

dill sprigs

Instructions

STEP 1

Put the butter, flour and milk in a pan and cook, stirring over the heat until thickened. Stir in the cheese, in small spoonfuls, and the dill; season to taste, then beat to incorporate.

STEP 2

Heat oven to 200C/180C fan/gas 6. Butter 6 x 150ml soufflé dishes and line the base with baking paper. Stir the egg yolks into the sauce, add the chopped salmon and lemon. Whisk the egg whites until stiff, then carefully fold into the salmon mix. Spoon into the dishes and bake in a tin half-filled with cold water for 15 mins until risen and golden. Cool; don't worry if they sink.

STEP 3

To freeze, cool completely, then overwrap the dishes with baking paper and foil. They will keep in the freezer for 6 weeks. Thaw for 5 hrs in the fridge.

STEP 4

When ready to serve, very carefully turn the soufflés out of their dishes, peel off the lining paper and place on squares of baking paper. Top with the crème fraîche and bake for 10-15 mins at 200C/180C fan/gas 6 until the soufflés start to puff up. Quickly top each with a frill of salmon and a dill sprig. Serve on their own or with some dressed salad leaves.

Stir-fried chicken with broccoli & brown rice

Ingredients

- 200g trimmed broccoli florets (about 6), halved

- 1 chicken breast (approx 180g), diced

- 15g ginger, cut into shreds

- 2 garlic cloves, cut into shreds

- 1 red onion, sliced

- 1 roasted red pepper, from a jar, cut into cubes

- 2 tsp olive oil

- 1 tsp mild chilli powder

- 1 tbsp reduced-salt soy sauce

- 1 tbsp honey

- 250g pack cooked brown rice

Instructions

- STEP 1

Put the kettle on to boil and tip the broccoli into a medium pan ready to go on the heat. Pour the water over the broccoli then boil for 4 mins.

- STEP 2

Heat the olive oil in a non-stick wok and stir-fry the ginger, garlic and onion for 2 mins, add the mild chilli powder and stir briefly. Add the chicken and stir-fry for 2 mins more. Drain the broccoli and reserve the water. Tip the broccoli into the wok with the soy, honey, red pepper and 4 tbsp broccoli water then cook until heated through. Meanwhile, heat the rice following the pack instructions and serve with the stir-fry.

Chicken & chorizo ragu

Ingredients

- 120g cooking chorizo, chopped

- 1 red onion, chopped

- 2 garlic cloves, grated

- 1 tsp hot smoked paprika

- 80g sundried tomatoes, roughly chopped

- 600g skinless and boneless chicken thighs

- 400g can chopped tomatoes

- 100ml chicken stock

- 1 lemon, juiced

- jacket potatoes, chopped parsley and soured cream, to serve (optional)

Instructions

- STEP 1

Fry the chorizo over a medium heat in a large saucepan or flameproof casserole dish for 5 mins or until it releases its oil and starts to char at the edges. Add the onion and fry for 5 mins more or until soft. Tip in the garlic and cook for 2 mins before stirring in the paprika and sundried tomatoes. Add the chicken thighs and fry for 2 mins each side until they are well coated in the spices and beginning to brown.

- STEP 2

Pour in the chopped tomatoes and stock, and turn the heat down. Cover and cook for 40 mins until the chicken is falling apart and the sauce is thick. Stir the lemon juice through. Serve by piling spoonfuls of the ragu into hot jacket potatoes with parsley sprinkled over and a dollop of soured cream, if you like.

Steaks with goulash sauce & sweet potato fries

Ingredients

- 3 tsp rapeseed oil, plus extra for the steaks

- 250g sweet potatoes, peeled and cut into narrow chips

- 1 tbsp fresh thyme leaves

- 2 small onions, halved and sliced (190g)

- 1 green pepper, deseeded and diced

- 2 garlic cloves, sliced

- 1 tsp smoked paprika

- 85g cherry tomatoes, halved

- 1 tbsp tomato purée

- 1 tsp vegetable bouillon powder

- 2 x 125g fillet steaks, rubbed with a little rapeseed oil

- 200g bag baby spinach, wilted in a pan or the microwave

Instructions

- STEP 1

Heat oven to 240C/220C fan/gas 7 and put a wire rack on top of a baking tray. Toss the sweet potatoes and thyme with 2 tsp oil in a bowl, then scatter them over the rack and set aside until ready to cook.

- STEP 2

Heat 1 tsp oil in a non-stick pan, add the onions, cover the pan and leave to cook for 5 mins. Take off the lid and stir – they should be a little charred now. Stir in the green pepper and garlic, cover the pan and cook for 5 mins more. Put the potatoes in the oven and bake for 15 mins.

- STEP 3

While the potatoes are cooking, stir the paprika into the onions and peppers, pour in 150ml water and stir in the cherry tomatoes, tomato purée and bouillon. Cover and simmer for 10 mins.

- STEP 4

Pan-fry the steak in a hot, non-stick pan for 2-3 mins each side depending on their thickness. Rest for 5 mins. Spoon the goulash sauce onto plates and top with the beef. Serve the chips and spinach alongside.

Minty griddled chicken & peach salad

Ingredients

- 1 lime, zested and juiced

- 1 tbsp rapeseed oil

- 2 tbsp mint, finely chopped, plus a few leaves to serve

- 1 garlic clove, finely grated

- 2 skinless chicken breast fillets (300g)

- 160g fine beans, trimmed and halved

- 2 peaches (200g), each cut into 8 thick wedges

- 1 red onion, cut into wedges

- 1 large Little Gem lettuce (165g), roughly shredded

- ½ x 60g pack rocket

- 1 small avocado, stoned and sliced

- 240g cooked new potatoes

Instructions

- STEP 1

Mix the lime zest and juice, oil and mint, then put half in a bowl with the garlic. Thickly slice the chicken at a slight angle, add to the garlic mixture and toss together with plenty of black pepper.

- STEP 2

Cook the beans in a pan of water for 3-4 mins until just tender. Meanwhile, griddle the chicken and onion for a few mins each side until cooked and tender. Transfer to a plate, then quickly griddle the peaches. If you don't have a griddle pan, use a non-stick frying pan with a drop of oil.

- STEP 3

Toss the warm beans and onion in the remaining mint mixture, and pile onto a platter or into individual shallow bowls with the lettuce and rocket. Top with the avocado, peaches and chicken and scatter over the mint. Serve with the potatoes while still warm.

Spinach kedgeree with spiced salmon

Ingredients

- 2 tsp rapeseed oil

- 1 large onion, halved and sliced

- thumb-sized piece of ginger, finely chopped

- ½ tsp cumin seeds

- ½ tsp ground cinnamon

- 6-8 cardamom pods, seeds crushed

- 1½ tsp ground turmeric

- 1½ tsp ground coriander

- 1 red chilli, deseeded and sliced

- 1 garlic clove, finely chopped

- 1 large red pepper, deseeded and roughly chopped

- 70g brown basmati rice

- 375ml vegetable stock, made with 2 tsp bouillon powder

- 160g baby spinach leaves, roughly chopped

For the salmon

- 3 tbsp fat-free natural yogurt

- 1 tbsp finely chopped mint or coriander

- 2 skinless wild salmon fillets

- 1 tbsp toasted almonds, to serve

Instructions

- STEP 1

Heat the oil in a large frying pan and fry the onion and ginger for 5 mins or until soft. Add the cumin, cinnamon, crushed cardamom seeds, and 1 tsp each of the turmeric and coriander. Cook for 30 secs until fragrant. Add the chilli, garlic, pepper and rice, stir briefly, then pour in the stock. Cover and simmer for 35 mins or until the rice is tender and the stock has been absorbed. If the rice is cooked but some liquid remains, remove the lid and simmer uncovered to allow the liquid to evaporate. Add the spinach, cover and cook for 3 mins to wilt.

- STEP 2

Meanwhile, prepare the salmon. Heat the grill to medium and line a baking sheet with foil. Mix the yogurt with the mint or coriander and the remaining turmeric and ground coriander. Spread the yogurt mixture over the salmon, then transfer to the prepared baking sheet and grill for 8-10 mins until the fish can be flaked easily with a fork. Top the kedgeree with the salmon fillets or flake the fish into it, and scatter over the almonds to serve.

Mustard salmon & veg bake with horseradish sauce

Ingredients

- 4 parsnips, sliced lengthways

- 4 small raw beetroot, thickly sliced

- 6 carrots, sliced lengthways

- 2 tbsp olive oil

- 4 x 125g/4½oz pieces salmon with skin

- 2 tbsp grainy mustard

- 2 tbsp hot horseradish

- 150ml crème fraîche

- 1 tbsp cider vinegar

- 1 tbsp chopped dill

How to Make

- STEP 1

Heat oven to 200C/180C fan/gas 6. Toss all the vegetables with the oil and season well. Spread in a single layer on 2 baking trays (or 1 very large tray) and roast for 30 mins.

- STEP 2

Season the salmon and spread over the mustard. In the final 10 mins of cooking the veg, add the salmon to the trays.

- STEP 3

In a small bowl, mix together the horseradish, crème fraîche, vinegar, dill and some seasoning. Serve the salmon with the sauce and veg.

Hake fish cakes with mustard middles

Ingredients

For the fish cakes

- 450g floury potatoes, cut into chunks (we used Rooster potatoes)

- 1 bay leaf

- a few peppercorns

- 450g skinless hake fillet, cut into 4

- bunch spring onions, finely shredded

- 1 whole nutmeg

- 3 tbsp plain flour, seasoned

- 1 egg

- 100g fresh breadcrumbs

- 2l vegetable oil, for deep-frying

- salad leaves, to serve

- lemon wedges, to serve

For the mustard middles

- 100g full-fat crème fraîche

- 50g strong cheddar, grated

- 1 egg yolk (reserve the white)

- 1 tbsp wholegrain mustard

How to Make

- STEP 1

Mix all the mustard middle Ingredients together. Drape cling film across a muffin tin, then spoon the mix into 4 of the wells. Freeze for 30 mins or until solid.

- STEP 2

Put the potatoes, bay leaf and peppercorns in a pan of cold water, bring to the boil and cook for 20 mins or until tender. Remove and allow to steam-dry in a colander. Add the fish to the water and simmer for 5 mins until it is just cooked through at the thickest part.

- STEP 3

Mash the potatoes and stir in the spring onions, a little freshly grated nutmeg and some seasoning. Drain the hake, then flake it into the mash. Gently mix everything together and leave to cool.

- STEP 4

Divide the fish mixture into 4. Shape 1 fish cake at a time, moulding it into a ball. Make a well in the centre of the ball and push a frozen mustard middle into it, then shape the mash around it to make a smooth hockey-puck shape. Repeat with the remaining fish, then freeze for 15 mins.

- STEP 5

Using 3 shallow bowls, add the flour to one; put the egg and reserved egg white in another, and the breadcrumbs in the third. Beat the eggs with some seasoning. Thoroughly coat the fishcakes first in the flour, then the egg , then the breadcrumbs. Freeze the fish cakes until firm. Can be frozen for up to 1 month – defrost in the fridge for 2 hrs before cooking.

- STEP 6

When ready to cook, heat the oil to 180C in a large, deep saucepan (or use a fat fryer) and the oven to 190C/170C fan/gas 5. Fry the fish cakes for 7 mins, turning halfway, until crisp. Drain on kitchen paper, transfer to a baking sheet and bake for 5 mins (15 mins from frozen) so the middles are hot. Serve with dressed leaves and a lemon wedge.

Baked sea bream with tomatoes & coriander

Ingredients

- 4 large potatoes, about 1kg/2lb 4oz

- 2 garlic cloves, finely chopped

- pinch dried chilli flakes

- pinch saffron

- 1 bunch coriander, roughly chopped

- 4 whole sea bream, cleaned and gutted

- 1 tbsp olive oil, plus extra for greasing

- juice 2 limes

- 125ml white wine

- handful sundried tomatoes

- handful pine nuts, toasted

- 4 thin slices pancetta or smoked streaky bacon

How to Make

- STEP 1

Heat the oven to 200C/180C fan/gas 6. Slice the potatoes thinly, put in a large saucepan and cover with cold salted water. Bring to the boil and drain, then lay onto the base of a lightly oiled large baking tray. Scatter over the garlic, chilli, saffron and a little of the coriander.

- STEP 2

Slash the fish through the flesh down to the bone – this allows it to cook evenly and quicker than normal. Season and rub with the olive oil. Lay the fish on the potatoes and top with the lime juice, wine, tomatoes and pine nuts. Lay the pancetta slices over the fish and bake for 20-25 mins or until the fish is cooked through. Check by pulling out one of the fins on the back, it should come away easily. Serve the fish scattered with the remaining coriander.

Herby fish fingers

Ingredients

- 50g crustless stale white bread

- finely grated zest of a large lemon

- 2 tbsp each roughly chopped fresh dill, fresh chives and fresh parsley

- 500g skinless lemon sole fillets

- 2 tbsp seasoned flour

- 1 egg, beaten

- vegetable oil, for shallow frying

How to Make

- STEP 1

Pulse the bread to coarse crumbs in the food processor. Add the lemon zest, herbs and a pinch of salt, and pulse to make bright green, fine breadcrumbs.

- STEP 2

Cut the lemon sole into thick strips, about 3 x 10cm. Dust each fish piece with the fl our, shake off any excess, then dip into the egg then the breadcrumbs. At this stage, they can be cooked straight away, kept in the fridge for a few hours, or frozen.

- STEP 3

To serve, heat about 1cm of oil in a large frying pan. Once it's nice and hot, fry the fish fingers a few at a time for 1-2 mins on each side. Drain on kitchen paper, and keep warm while you continue with the rest. When they are all cooked, serve straight away with the oven-roasted chips and tartare sauce.

Salmon & lemon mini fish cakes

Ingredients

- 2 large baking potatoes

- 2 tbsp olive oil

- grated zest and juice ½ lemon

- 1 egg yolk

- 140g smoked salmon trimmings, plus extra to serve

- 1 tbsp chopped parsley, plust extra

- 2 tbsp gluten-free flour mixed with 1 tsp coarsely ground pepper

- a little oil, for frying

How to Make

- STEP 1

Microwave potatoes on high for 10 mins until tender. Leave to cool for 5 mins, scoop the flesh in a bowl, then mash and leave to cool. Season with olive oil, lemon zest and juice to taste, then mix in the egg, salmon and parsley. Shape into small rounds 3cm wide and 1cm deep. Chill for 15 mins.

- STEP 2

Dust each cake with the peppered flour, then fry over a low heat in a little oil for 2-3 mins on each side. Drain on kitchen paper and serve garnished with salmon and parsley.

SOUP RECIPES FOR VITILIGO

Corn & split pea chowder

Ingredients

200g dried yellow split peas

3 celery sticks (about 160g), sliced

1 thyme sprig, plus 1 tbsp thyme leaves

2 onions (350g), halved and sliced

1 tbsp rapeseed oil

50g ginger, finely grated

2 red chillies, deseeded and sliced

3 garlic cloves, chopped

1 large green pepper, chopped into small pieces

1 potato (about 215g), unpeeled, cut into 1-2cm pieces

2 tbsp vegetable bouillon powder

320g frozen sweetcorn

150g coconut yogurt

Instructions

STEP 1

Tip the split peas, celery and thyme sprig into a medium pan with 1 litre of boiling water, bring back to the boil and simmer, covered, for 25 mins.

STEP 2

Meanwhile, fry the onion in the oil in a large pan for 10 mins. Stir in the ginger, chilli and garlic. Tip in the pepper and potato, and pour in ½ litre boiling water with the bouillon and remaining thyme. Tip in the split pea mixture and corn, bring to the boil, then cover and simmer for 30-35 mins until the veg is tender.

STEP 3

Remove the thyme sprig. Take out a third of the veg, then purée the rest in the pan with a hand blender (or use a potato masher). Return the veg to the pan with the yogurt, and stir well.

Broccoli and kale green soup

Ingredients

500ml stock, made by mixing 1 tbsp bouillon powder and boiling water in a jug

1 tbsp sunflower oil

2 garlic cloves, sliced

thumb-sized piece ginger, sliced

½ tsp ground coriander

3cm/1in piece fresh turmeric root, peeled and grated, or 1/2 tsp ground turmeric

pinch of pink Himalayan salt

200g courgettes, roughly sliced

85g broccoli

100g kale, chopped

1 lime, zested and juiced

small pack parsley, roughly chopped, reserving a few whole leaves to serve

Instructions

STEP 1

Put the oil in a deep pan, add the garlic, ginger, coriander, turmeric and salt, fry on a medium heat for 2 mins, then add 3 tbsp water to give a bit more moisture to the spices.

STEP 2

Add the courgettes, making sure you mix well to coat the slices in all the spices, and continue cooking for 3 mins. Add 400ml stock and leave to simmer for 3 mins.

STEP 3

Add the broccoli, kale and lime juice with the rest of the stock. Leave to cook again for another 3-4 mins until all the vegetables are soft.

STEP 4

Take off the heat and add the chopped parsley. Pour everything into a blender and blend on high speed until smooth. It will be a beautiful green with bits of dark speckled through (which is the kale). Garnish with lime zest and parsley.

Fresh tomato soup with cheesy cornbread

Ingredients

For the bread

40g wholemeal self-raising flour

85g ground polenta

1 tsp baking powder

40g mature cheddar, finely grated

1 tsp smoked paprika

3 spring onions (35g), finely sliced

1 green chilli, deseeded, finely sliced

1 large egg

125ml milk

For the soup

2 tsp rapeseed oil

3-5 sticks celery (165g), finely chopped

2 onions, chopped

4 carrots (320g), diced

325g floury potatoes, grated

500g tomatoes, chopped

4 tsp vegetable bouillon powder made up to 1 1/2 litre with boiling water

3 tbsp tomato purée

2 large garlic cloves, finely grated

flat-leaf parsley, chopped, to serve

Instructions

STEP 1

First, make the bread. Heat oven to 200C/180C fan/gas 6 and line the base of a non-stick 500g loaf tin with baking parchment. Tip the flour, polenta and baking powder into a bowl with half the cheese, the paprika, onions and chilli, then toss together. Add the egg and milk and mix well. Turn out into the tin and top with the remaining cheese. Bake for 20-25 mins until golden and a skewer inserted into the centre comes out clean.

STEP 2

To make the soup, heat the oil in a large pan and fry the celery, onion and carrots for 10 mins until softened. Add the potatoes, tomatoes, bouillon, tomato purée and garlic, then stir well. Cover with a lid and cook for 20 mins.

STEP 3

Remove from the heat and blitz until smooth with a hand blender.

Summer pistou

Ingredients

1 tbsp rapeseed oil

2 leeks, finely sliced

1 large courgette, finely diced

1l boiling vegetable stock (made from scratch or with reduced-salt bouillon)

400g can cannellini or haricot beans, drained

200g green beans, chopped

3 tomatoes, chopped

3 garlic cloves, finely chopped

small pack basil

40g freshly grated parmesan

Instructions

STEP 1

Heat the oil in a large pan and fry the leeks and courgette for 5 mins to soften. Pour in the stock, add three-quarters of the haricot beans with the green beans, half the tomatoes, and simmer for 5-8 mins until the vegetables are tender.

STEP 2

Meanwhile, blitz the remaining beans and tomatoes, the garlic and basil in a food processor (or in a bowl with a stick blender) until smooth, then stir in the Parmesan. Stir the sauce into the soup, cook for 1 min, then ladle half into bowls or pour into a flask for a packed lunch. Chill the remainder. Will keep for a couple of days.

Spinach soup

Ingredients

25g butter

1 bunch spring onions, chopped

1 leek (about 120g), sliced

2 small sticks celery (about 85g), sliced

1 small potato (about 200g), peeled and diced

½ tsp ground black pepper

1l stock (made with two chicken or vegetable stock cubes)

2 x 200-235g bags spinach

150g half-fat crème fraîche

Instructions

STEP 1

Heat the butter in a large saucepan. Add the spring onions, leek, celery and potato. Stir and put on the lid. Sweat for 10 minutes, stirring a couple of times.

STEP 2

Pour in the stock and cook for 10 – 15 minutes until the potato is soft.

STEP 3

Add the spinach and cook for a couple of minutes until wilted. Use a hand blender to blitz to a smooth soup.

STEP 4

Stir in the crème fraîche. Reheat and serve.

Red lentil soup

Ingredients

1 white onion, finely sliced

2 tsp olive oil

3 garlic cloves, sliced

2 carrots, scrubbed and diced

85g red lentils

1 vegetable stock cube, crumbled

generous sprigs parsley, chopped (about 2 tbsp) plus a few extra leaves

Instructions

STEP 1

Put the kettle on to boil while you finely slice the onion. Heat the oil in a medium pan, add the onion and fry for 2 mins while you slice the garlic and dice the carrots. Add them to the pan, and cook briefly over the heat.

STEP 2

Pour in 1 litre of the boiling water from the kettle, stir in the lentils and stock cube, then cover the pan and cook over a medium heat for 15 mins until the lentils are tender. Take off the heat and stir in the parsley. Ladle into bowls, and scatter with extra parsley leaves, if you like.

Courgette, pea & pesto soup

Ingredients

1 tbsp olive oil

1 garlic clove, sliced

500g courgettes, quartered lengthways and chopped

200g frozen peas

400g can cannellini beans, drained and rinsed

1l hot vegetable stock

2 tbsp basil pesto, or vegetarian alternative

Instructions

STEP 1

Heat the oil in a large saucepan. Cook the garlic for a few seconds, then add the courgettes and cook for 3 mins until they start to soften. Stir in the peas and cannellini beans, pour on the hot stock and cook for a further 3 mins.

STEP 2

Stir the pesto through the soup with some seasoning, then ladle into bowls and serve with crusty brown bread, if you like. Or pop in a flask to take to work.

Broccoli & stilton soup

Ingredients

2 tbsp rapeseed oil

1 onion, finely chopped

1 stick celery, sliced

1 leek, sliced

1 medium potato, diced

1 knob butter

1l low salt or homemade chicken or vegetable stock

1 head broccoli, roughly chopped

140g stilton, or other blue cheese, crumbled

Instructions

STEP 1

Heat 2 tbsp rapeseed oil in a large saucepan and then add 1 finely chopped onion. Cook on a medium heat until soft. Add a splash of water if the onion starts to catch.

STEP 2

Add 1 sliced celery stick, 1 sliced leek, 1 diced medium potato and a knob of butter. Stir until melted, then cover with a lid. Allow to sweat for 5 minutes then remove the lid.

STEP 3

Pour in 1l of chicken or vegetable stock and add any chunky bits of stalk from 1 head of broccoli. Cook for 10-15 minutes until all the vegetables are soft.

STEP 4

Add the rest of the roughly chopped broccoli and cook for a further 5 minutes.

STEP 5

Carefully transfer to a blender and blitz until smooth.

STEP 6

Stir in 140g crumbled stilton, allowing a few lumps to remain. Season with black pepper and serve.

Chicken & sweetcorn soup

Ingredients

1 chicken carcass

4 thin slices fresh ginger, plus 1 tbsp finely grated

2 onions, quartered

3 garlic cloves, finely grated

2 tsp apple cider vinegar

325g can sweetcorn

3 spring onions, whites thinly sliced, greens sliced at an angle

100g cooked chicken, shredded

2 tsp tamari

2 eggs, beaten

few drops sesame oil, to serve (optional)

Instructions

STEP 1

Boil a large kettle of water. Break the carcass into a big non-stick pan and add the ginger slices, onion and two-thirds of the garlic. Cook, stirring, for about 2 mins – the meat will stick to the base of the pan, but this will add to the flavour. Pour in 1.5 litres of boiling water, stir in the vinegar, then cover and simmer for 2 hrs.

STEP 2

Put a large sieve over a bowl and pour through the contents of the pan. Measure the liquid in the bowl – you want around 450ml. If you have too much, return to the pan and boil with the lid off to reduce it. Transfer the onion from the sieve to a bowl with three-quarters of the sweetcorn. Blitz until smooth with a hand blender.

STEP 3

Return the broth to the pan, and tip in the puréed corn, remaining sweetcorn and garlic, the grated ginger, the whites of the spring onions and the chicken. Simmer for 5 mins, then stir in the tamari. Turn off the heat, and quickly drizzle in the egg, stirring a little to create egg threads. Season with pepper, then ladle into the bowls. Top with the spring onion greens and a few drops of sesame oil, if using.

Moroccan spiced cauliflower & almond soup

Ingredients

1 large cauliflower

2 tbsp olive oil

½ tsp each ground cinnamon, cumin and coriander

2 tbsp harissa paste, plus extra drizzle

1l hot vegetable or chicken stock

50g toasted flaked almond, plus extra to serve

Instructions

STEP 1

Cut the cauliflower into small florets. Fry olive oil, ground cinnamon, cumin and coriander and harissa paste for 2 mins in a large pan. Add the cauliflower, stock and almonds. Cover and cook for 20 mins until the cauliflower is tender. Blend soup until smooth, then serve with an extra drizzle of harissa and a sprinkle of toasted almonds.

Leek, fennel & potato soup with cashel blue cheese

Ingredients

2 heads fennel

3 large leeks, trimmed, washed and finely sliced

60g butter

1 large potato, peeled and diced

900ml chicken stock or water

1 garlic clove, sliced

100ml double cream

50g walnuts, toasted

75g Cashel Blue cheese, crumbled

Instructions

STEP 1

Quarter the fennel and discard the tough outer leaves and the hard core from each piece. Slice the rest of the flesh, including any little fronds.

STEP 2

Heat the butter in a saucepan and add the fennel, leeks and potato. Cook over a medium heat for about 5 mins, turning the vegetables over in the butter. The vegetables shouldn't colour. Add a splash of water, cover the pan and cook the vegetables for 20 mins, stirring every so often. Add the stock or water and garlic, season, bring to the boil, then turn the heat down low and cover the pan with a lid or foil.

STEP 3

Cook for about 10-15 mins, until everything is completely tender. Stir in the cream and leave to cool. Purée in a blender until completely smooth. Check the seasoning and return the mixture to the saucepan – you can reheat it quickly just before serving. Ladle into bowls and scatter each one with the walnuts and cheese.

Smoky tomato, chipotle & charred corn soup

Ingredients

1 tbsp rapeseed oil

1 onion, finely chopped

2 garlic cloves, chopped

2 tsp ground coriander

small bunch of coriander, stalks chopped and leaves left whole

400g can chopped tomatoes

600ml vegetable stock

1-1½ tbsp chipotle chilli paste

2 corn on the cobs

50g feta, crumbled

4 tbsp fat-free Greek yogurt

Instructions

STEP 1

Heat the oil in a casserole dish and fry the onion for 10 mins until beginning to soften. Add the garlic, ground coriander and coriander stalks, and cook for 1 min. Stir though the tomatoes, stock and chipotle and bring to a simmer. Cook, covered, over a low heat for 20 mins, stirring occasionally.

STEP 2

Meanwhile, bring a pan of water to the boil and cook the corn for 4 mins. Drain and leave to cool a little. Cut the kernels off the cob with a sharp knife. Heat a non-stick frying pan over a high heat. Add the corn and fry for 5-7 mins or until charred, stirring now and again.

Creamy pumpkin & lentil soup

Ingredients

1 tbsp olive oil, plus 1 tsp

2 onions, chopped

2 garlic cloves, chopped

approx 800g chopped pumpkin flesh, plus the seeds

100g split red lentil

½ small pack thyme, leaves picked, plus extra to serve

1l hot vegetable stock

pinch of salt and sugar

50g crème fraîche, plus extra to serve

Instructions

STEP 1

Heat the oil in a large pan. Fry the onions until softened and starting to turn golden. Stir in the garlic, pumpkin flesh, lentils and thyme, then pour in the hot stock. Season, cover and simmer for 20-25 mins until the lentils and vegetables are tender.

STEP 2

Meanwhile, wash the pumpkin seeds. Remove any flesh still clinging to them, then dry them with kitchen paper. Heat the 1 tsp oil in a non-stick pan and fry the seeds until they start to jump and pop. Stir frequently, but cover the pan in between to keep them in it. When the seeds look nutty and toasted, add a sprinkling of salt and a pinch of sugar, and stir well.

Chorizo & chickpea soup

Ingredients

400g can chopped tomato

110g pack of chorizo sausage (unsliced)

140g wedge Savoy cabbage

sprinkling dried chilli flakes

410g can chickpea, drained and rinsed

1 chicken or vegetable stock cube

crusty bread or garlic bread, to serve

Instructions

STEP 1

Put a medium pan on the heat and tip in the tomatoes, followed by a can of water. While the tomatoes are heating, quickly chop the chorizo into chunky pieces (removing any skin) and shred the cabbage.

STEP 2

Pile the chorizo and cabbage into the pan with the chilli flakes and chickpeas, then crumble in the stock cube. Stir well, cover and leave to bubble over a high heat for 6 mins or until the cabbage is just tender. Ladle into bowls and eat with crusty or garlic bread.

White velvet soup with smoky almonds

Ingredients

2 tsp rapeseed oil

2 large garlic cloves, sliced

2 leeks, trimmed so they're mostly white in colour, washed well, then sliced (about 240g)

200g cauliflower, chopped

2 tsp vegetable bouillon powder

400g cannellini beans, rinsed

fresh nutmeg, for grating

100ml whole milk

25g whole almonds, chopped

½ tsp smoked paprika

2 x 25g slices rye bread, to serve

Instructions

STEP 1

Heat the oil in a large pan. Add the garlic, leeks and cauliflower and cook for about 5 mins, stirring frequently, until starting to soften (but not colouring).

STEP 2

Stir in the vegetable bouillon and beans, pour in 600ml boiling water and add a few generous gratings of the nutmeg. Cover and leave to simmer for 15 mins until the leeks and cauliflower are tender. Add the milk and blitz with a hand blender until smooth and creamy.

STEP 3

Put the almonds in a dry pan and cook very gently for 1 min, or until toasted, then remove from the heat. Scatter the paprika over the almonds and mix well. Ladle the soup into bowls, top with the spicy nuts and serve with the rye bread.

PART V

LIFESTYLE TIPS AND ADDITIONAL CONSIDERATIONS

If you have vitiligo, the following self-care tactics may help you care for your skin and improve its appearance:

• **Protect your skin from the sun and artificial sources of UV light.** Use a broad-spectrum, water-resistant sunscreen with an SPF of at least 30. Apply sunscreen generously and reapply every two hours — or more often if you're swimming or sweating.

You can also seek shade and wear clothing that shields your skin from the sun. Don't use tanning beds and sunlamps.

Protecting your skin from the sun helps prevent sunburn of the discolored skin. Sunscreen also minimizes tanning, which accentuates the vitiligo patches.

- **Conceal affected skin.** Makeup and self-tanning products can help minimize the differences in skin color. You may need to try several brands of makeup or self-tanners to find one that blends well with your normal skin tone. The coloring of self-tanning products doesn't wash off, but it gradually fades over several days. If you use a self-tanner, select one that contains dihydroxyacetone, as it is approved by the U.S. Food and Drug Administration.

- **Don't get a tattoo.** Damage to your skin, such as that caused by a tattoo, may cause a new patch of vitiligo to appear within two weeks.

Alternative medicine

Limited studies show that the herb Ginkgo biloba may return skin color in people with vitiligo. Other small studies show that alpha-lipoic acid, folic acid, vitamin C and vitamin B-12 plus phototherapy may restore skin color for some people.

As with any nonprescription treatment, check with your health care provider before trying alternative medicine therapies to be sure they won't interfere with other treatments you're using.

Coping and support

The change in your appearance caused by vitiligo might make you feel stressed, self-conscious or sad. These self-care approaches can help you cope with vitiligo:

- **Make a good connection.** Find a doctor who knows a lot about the condition. A dermatologist is a doctor who specializes in the care of skin.

- **Learn about your condition.** Find out as much as you can about vitiligo and your treatment options so that you can help decide what steps to take.

- **Communicate your feelings.** Let your health care provider know if you're feeling depressed. You might benefit from a referral to a mental health provider who specializes in helping people with depression.

- **Talk with others.** Ask your health care provider about psychotherapy or support groups in your area for people with vitiligo.

- **Confide in loved ones.** Seek understanding and support from your family and friends.

www.ingramcontent.com/pod-product-compliance
Lightning Source LLC
Chambersburg PA
CBHW071826210526
45479CB00001B/13